Bizarre behaviours

Human behaviour, which holds a fascination for most people, can best be viewed as lying on a spectrum – from 'normality' at one end to extreme deviation at the other, with obvious grey areas in between. Even the most deviant-seeming behaviours appear to have their counterparts in 'normality', and such behaviours can often be explained (at least in part) when viewed in their socio-cultural and psychological contexts.

In *Bizarre Behaviours* the author examines a selection of such behaviours, the aim being to show their diversity and to offer an introduction to the wide range of departure from human normality. In doing so, he considers some of the less well-known psychiatric syndromes, some disorders that are said to be culturally determined, and conditions which cross the boundaries between psychiatric and religious explanation. He also gives particular attention to one extreme form of deviation – vampirism, since in his view it demonstrates very clearly the need for a multi-disciplinary approach to explanation.

There are very few books which deal with the topics discussed and, although there are hundreds of papers in a wide range of journals, some of these are not easily accessible to the professional worker, and are even less accessible to the general reader. *Bizarre Behaviours* brings together some of this less readily available literature and synthesizes it, enabling the book to be read on two levels. It may be read by anyone interested in acquiring a general over-view of the topic and the more specialist reader will find the extensive notes and references useful for further exploration.

Bizarre Behaviours will be of value to all who have to confront behaviour that often appears to be incomprehensible (and sometimes frightening). These include psychiatrists, psychologists, social workers, penal staff, the police, general practitioners, the clergy of all denominations, lawyers, and sentencers. The work will also have a fascination for the interested general reader who is keen to know more about the origins and infinite variety of human behaviour.

Herschel Prins has had nearly forty years' experience of working with, and teaching about, socially and psychologically disturbed individuals. Since retiring from the Directorship of the School of Social Work at Leicester University, he has lectured and acted as a consultant on social aspects of forensic psychiatry and on clinical criminology. He is a member of the Mental Health Review Tribunal and has been a member of the Parole Board and of the Mental Health Act Commission.

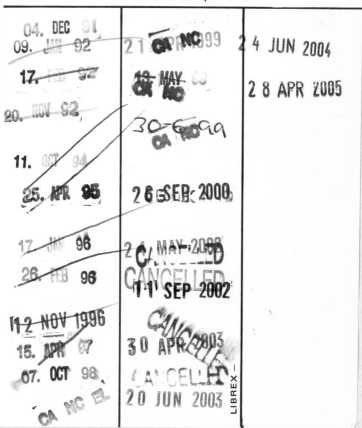

Bizarre behaviours
Boundaries of psychiatric disorder

Herschel Prins

Foreword by Dr Murray Cox

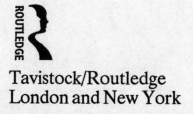

Tavistock/Routledge
London and New York

First published 1990
by Routledge
11 New Fetter Lane, London EC4P 4EE

Simultaneously published in the USA and Canada
by Routledge
a division of Routledge, Chapman and Hall, Inc.
29 West 35th Street, New York, NY 10001

Typeset by NWL Editorial Services, Langport, Somerset TA10 9DG
Printed and bound in Great Britain by
Biddles Ltd, Guildford and King's Lynn

British Library Cataloguing in Publication Data
Prins, Herschel A. (Herschel Albert), *1928–*
    Bizarre behaviours. Boundaries of psychiatric disorder.
    1. Man. Mental disorders
    I. Title
    616.89

Library of Congress Cataloging in Publication Data
Prins, Herschel A.
    Bizarre behaviours/Herschel Prins
    p.   cm.
    Includes bibliographical references.
    1. Deviant behavior.   I. Title.
    HM291.P72   1990   90–32965
    302.5'42—dc20   CIP

ISBN 0–415–01835–8
ISBN 0–415–01836–6 (pbk)

Parry 6802 / 10.99. 8.91

This book is dedicated with affection and respect to my many psychiatrist friends and colleagues in the hope that they will continue to show me the kind indulgence they have done in the past.

'Blessed art thou, O Lord, Our God,
King of the Universe, who hath
Made a distinction between sacred and profane;
Between light and darkness.'

(Prayer at the service for Passover,
from the *Haggadah*)

Contents

Acknowledgements

In order to produce this book, I have had to encompass many disciplines, some more familiar to me than others. I hope that experts in any of these disciplines will bear with me if at any point I have misrepresented their findings or views; I have endeavoured to be as accurate in my researches as possible. To these many writers I owe an enormous debt and I record it here. A great many people responded to my enquiries in connection with the material on vampirism in Chapter five. I am most grateful to them for their ready assistance and to those correspondents who have continued to furnish me with interesting data since the original research was undertaken. This is the fourth book I have written for Tavistock Publications (now Routledge). The editorial staff of that house have been unfailingly helpful in their support, advice and encouragement over the years. I owe a special debt of gratitude to Gill Davies for her support in the early days of our association, and to Gordon Smith, Caroline Lane and Edwina Welham during the last ten years. The work of an author is heavily dependent upon skilled secretarial assistance. Once again, I have been most ably served by Janet Kirkwood who, despite an increasingly busy professional and domestic life, has managed to make sense of my drafts, to spot errors, and to meet deadlines with good grace. Authors are also heavily dependent upon the support and tolerance of their families and I am no exception. My wife, Norma, has put up yet again with my absences and preoccupations with investigations that have encompassed a great deal of unusual and occasionally unpleasant material. She has accepted all this with good grace and in addition has read every word of the final manuscript. Any success that this book has as a literary offering owes much to her many judicious suggestions concerning grammar and style. My debt to all who have helped in the production of this book is considerable and any pleasure I may derive from its success will, I hope, be theirs also.

Foreword

Dr Murray Cox

> 'Now could I drink hot blood,
> And do such bitter business as the day
> Would quake to look on.'
>
> (*Hamlet*, Act III, Scene ii)

This book is primarily concerned with bizarre *behaviour*; not with bizarre experience. Its focus is the act; which may, or may not, be the acting-out of intrapsychic conflict. But precisely because behaviour can be a consequence of previous bizarre fantasy, those who work with patients having a bizarre fantasy-life are kept constantly on the alert. They need to distinguish metaphorical from concrete referents. Even our everyday language is permeated by metaphorical statements, such as 'I could torture you. And I mean it.' This may only imply 'I will hide your favourite chocolates'; though, in forensic experience, it may connote a prelude to savage physical and/or psychological mutilation. This diversity of possible connotations means that such behaviour cannot be divorced from the study of those inner world phenomena which may precede bizarre action, though they do not necessarily cause it.

The passage from *Hamlet* is usually taken to be a metaphorical statement. It conveys the intensity of the driving force behind Hamlet's yearning for homicidal revenge. And, though he is often accused of initial ambivalence, introspective procrastination and even of being preoccupied with blood, I have never heard of 'Hamlet the vampire' on the grounds that he could 'drink hot blood'. Nevertheless, rare though it is, vampirism is an established clinical syndrome. And, as such – sooner or later – it is very likely to be encountered within the field of forensic psychiatry and its cognate disciplines.

Herschel Prins, the author, has brought together a representative range of 'bizarre behaviours'. They extend from socially harmless deviations from the norm, to those extremities exemplified by the disturbed and sought by the vicariously prurient. He wisely preempts the predictable criticism that the topics chosen are capriciously selected. The professional, even if he works in a specialist setting in which rarities congregate, can never have sufficiently wide firsthand experience. And he, like the general reader who needs to be informed, will welcome this book which culls expertise from a diversity of disciplines and a variety of views.

Bizarre behaviour demands our most rigorous attention if we are to understand it, with a view to treating and, maybe, even preventing it. Yet there is a danger that conceptual categories collapse when our patient's behaviour baffles us; so that an amalgam of the analytic, behaviouristic and organic aetiologies does little more than hint at satisfactory explanatory hypotheses. Conceptual confusion may result at this point. We then risk reifying words from *Macbeth*: 'Confusion now hath made his masterpiece' (Act II, Scene iii). This transpires when we hear remarks such as 'This man is neither psychotic nor a psychopath. He's just evil.' Category derailment of this kind leads nowhere. An entirely different frame of reference is necessary if we are to invoke the category of evil. The discussion then becomes, 'There is evil in all of us. What form does it take in him? In you? In me?' A topic such as vampirism tends to polarise the interest, even of the best intentioned. We either distance ourselves, because – in more than one sense – it is unpalatable; and in any case, it is exceedingly rare. Or, we become pathologically over-interested. Either way, we then block the possibility of that informed discretionary judgement, which is so necessary for both diagnostic dynamic appraisal, and that balanced hovering attentiveness, which is the *sine qua non* of dynamic psychotherapy.

'Courageous' is not too strong a word to describe the author's attempt to explore several species of bizarre behaviours, which do not fall neatly within the safe confines of a single professional discipline. And this remains true, no matter whether we think of psychiatry, psychology, philosophy, sociology, anthropology, or theology.

I found myself wondering why most of my thoughts centred upon the relatively uncommon phenomenon of vampirism. But, on reflection, I think this proclivity is because the topic so well stresses the importance of distinguishing the metaphorical from the concrete implications of intended action. The individual-yet-generic example from *Hamlet* illustrates the point. After all, soon after saying 'Now I could drink hot blood', Hamlet – alone on the stage – and shortly to confront his mother, says 'I will speak daggers to her but use none' (*Hamlet*, Act III, Scene ii).

Because 'unusual behaviour' is an umbrella term, and a large one at that, this relatively slim volume implies that the author must have been rigorously selective, in order to deal in depth with even a few of his chosen topics. But this does not diminish the importance of the book for those who may encounter patients whose behaviour is 'bizarre'. This may occur at any moment; though, by the law of averages, it will probably take place when the worker is least prepared.

The huge topic of sexual deviation is not tackled systematically. Other books do that.[1] But there is sufficient material to remind the reader of the potentially polymorphic perversity of sexual activity. The author refers to 'bestiality'; though such deviation occurs at some point along the continuum of zoophilia, which ranges from marginally 'normal' caressing behaviour involving domestic pets, to the deviant extreme of necrophilia. I recall a patient saying 'I fucked a calf. But I killed it first.' The psychopathology implicit in such a brief statement is psychoanalytically condensed and existentially massive.

The book invites us to think about things which we may usually prefer to ignore, unless salacious hyper-interest has blurred our vision and unsettled our thought. It reminds us that many forms of bizarre behaviour are culture-bound. Perhaps this could be summarised by adopting the phrase of Kleinman's about the importance of 'the final common pathway'.[2] This concept is the result of many aetiological and cultural considerations. And, in terms of metaphorical or concrete sexual implications, 'the final common pathway' is capacious in its significance. There is the aetiological final common path. And there is the genital tract itself, as an anatomical 'final common path' – except for the non-genitally-oriented sexual deviant.

Bizarre Behaviours is provocative in the best sense. It provokes some difficult questions. It makes me ask myself 'Presuming that the professional worker needs to be informed about behaviour as bizarre as vampirism, how would I have written about it? What style would I choose to say what needs to be said, without being too dramatic, so as to appear voyeuristic, on the one hand, or too arid and detached, so as to appear defensive, on the other?'

Herschel Prins has asked himself these questions and tried to answer them. This book is the result. He is to be congratulated on achieving a balanced presentation of a theme that is fraught with pitfalls. But, when all is said and done and written, I cannot keep the words of Rabkin from my mind. He is commenting on Macbeth, surely a candidate for selection amongst those who exhibit bizarre behaviour: 'The understanding of character suggested by *Macbeth* is only secondarily psychoanalytic; more important is the implication that ultimate motivation is often crucially obscure ...'.[3]

Murray Cox MA DPM FRCPsych
Consultant Psychotherapist, Broadmoor Hospital;
Honorary Consultant Psychotherapist,
Inner London Probation Service;
Honorary Research Fellow, The Shakespeare Institute,
Stratford-upon-Avon (University of Birmingham)

References

1. I. Rosen (ed.), *Sexual Deviation* (2nd edn), London, Oxford University Press, 1979.
2. A. Kleinman, 'Anthropology and Psychiatry: The Role of Culture in Cross-cultural Research on Illness', *British Journal of Psychiatry*, 1987, vol. 151, pp. 447–454.
3. N. Rabkin, *Shakespeare and the Problem of Meaning*, Chicago, University of Chicago Press, 1981.

Chapter one

Context and purpose

'Behold I tell you a mystery.'
(I *Corinthians* 15: 51–52)

At around lunch-time on Wednesday, 19 August 1987, the normal affairs of the small country town of Hungerford were shattered by the apparent random shooting of fifteen people by gunman Michael Ryan; as is now well known, Ryan eventually turned his gun upon himself with fatal effect. Numerous people, including psychiatric experts, were quick to come forward and proffer explanations for his bizarre act of mayhem. According to some newspaper accounts one psychiatrist went so far as to suggest (without apparently ever having met Ryan) that he was likely to have been suffering from a schizophrenic illness since, in the course of his murderous activities, he had killed his mother. (It is of course true that matricide is sometimes committed by people suffering from schizophrenia, but people kill their mothers for a number of other reasons.) It is also worth making the point that the relationship between mental illness and violent crime is at best equivocal. From the brief accounts given of Ryan at the inquest, it would be extremely difficult to form an opinion as to what had motivated him or triggered off his orgy of killing. However, he was seen as someone who seemed to possess a single-minded preoccupation with firearms and their use, and it was said that he had tended to boast about his expertise in this field. There was also some suggestion that he lived in a phantasy world, but this was never substantiated. No satisfactory explanation has currently emerged for Ryan's behaviour.[1] However, speculation has raged, as it always does whenever we wish to try to explain and classify behaviour that appears to be bizarre, 'out of this world', and often terrifying. We have a need to bring order out of chaos and to derive comfort from trying to exercise control over that which seems uncontrollable. Some would say of Ryan (and many others before him) that he had run

1

'amok' (alternative spellings are *amuk, amuck*) but, as I shall show subsequently, this is a term best reserved for very specific forms of behaviour. On some occasions attempts have been made to explain the behaviour of people like Ryan who commit sudden mass killings or numerous killings over a long period of time (serial killings) on psychiatric or neurological grounds. It must be admitted that in many of these cases the behaviour defies this form of conclusive explanation.[2]

Elsewhere in this book I shall refer to a number of other forms of behaviour that appear to us to be bizarre and beyond immediate comprehension. For example, the person who repeatedly has himself or herself admitted to hospital for entirely unnecessary and often painful and intrusive surgical explorations and procedures; the individual who is only able to obtain sexual satisfaction when it is attempted under highly unusual conditions (such as with a dead body); the person who has a long-standing and quite unshakeable irrational belief that their spouse is being unfaithful; individuals who have a morbid desire to obtain and/or imbibe the blood of others; individuals who feel they are 'possessed'. These are just a selection of some of the behaviours I shall attempt to describe in this book. The choice is highly selective and some I have not described might well have been included; indeed, the choice is to a large extent idiosyncratic and may well be criticised on these grounds. In addition, some may consider that the material is not only partial, but too sensational, self-indulgent, voyeuristic or downright prurient. My defence to such possible accusations is two-fold. First, it would have been impossible to have included every type of bizarre behaviour within the confines of a short book. It is my aim to give the reader an introduction to some of these behaviours as indicators of the wide range of human departure from so-called normality. Second, in making my selection and in the manner in which I present it, I hope to alert my readers to the uncomfortable probability that these apparent extremes of behaviour may be but extensions of conduct that is, in fact, fairly universal. It is my contention that if we can recognise this, we may also learn a good deal about behaviour that we generally regard as normal. As in many areas of knowledge, it is often productive to move from the specific to the general in the search for enlightenment. As to claims that I may be playing into the hands of the prurient and the voyeuristic, I maintain that there are elements of both these phenomena in all of us and the sooner this is recognised the better. For in doing so, we may then be able better to understand those in whom the tendency seems to have gone beyond the bounds of the acceptable. I am also of the opinion that it is very easy for us to believe that it is always *others* who are besieged by forces that we do not understand; it is much harder to acknowledge that *we too* are often besieged and haunted by our own 'devils'. If this be so, then it renders us at best uncomprehending of the ills and fears of others and at worst makes us condemnatory and punitive towards them. It is my earnest hope that the accounts given in this book will enable readers to acknowledge in themselves what Carl Jung once described as our 'shadow' or 'dark' side.[3] Jung's work also alerts us to the powerful role of symbols and symbolism in our lives, phenomena as diverse as the mystical elements of the Kabbalah on the one hand and the Tarot on the other.[4] I shall refer to symbolic elements again when I consider the powerful significance of blood and other body fluids in connection with their association with certain manifestations of bizarre behaviour. At this point it is worth stressing that deviations from the so-called normal, even in comparatively mild form, must be seen in a socio-cultural context. For example, it was only a quarter of a century ago that we ceased to prescribe legal punishment for acts of homosexuality between adult consenting males in private. Up till then, apart from those involved in bringing about pressure for change, society at large had been perfectly happy for a comparatively mild form of deviation to be punished severely and for such offenders to suffer public disgrace and humiliation. There are, of course, large numbers of people today who consider that it was a retrograde step to reform the law in this fashion and who continue to regard deviant sexuality as both sinful and illegal. Another illustration may be found in what has usually been regarded as a late nineteenth-century disease – anorexia nervosa. Although it does not seem to have been described clinically before the late nineteenth century, it would appear to have a much longer history than this. Some authorities have cited as evidence of this the anorexic behaviour of certain holy women in mediaeval Italy. These women spent their lives starving, purging and punishing themselves in order to achieve a state of purity and grace. However, it has been shown that, to infuse their behaviour with real meaning, it must be examined against the background of the times in which they lived; bizarre though their behaviour may have appeared, it cannot be explained entirely in psychopathological terms. These women were trying to find a place and a role for themselves in a male-dominated religious and social hierarchy; and in order to achieve the highly prized state of holiness they had to adopt severe measures.[5]

There are, of course, other dimensions to my field of study. Although culture and milieu are vitally important, as are specific states of mind, there are certain purely physical, physiological and organic factors that may have an important bearing upon behaviour, adjudged to be strange or bizarre. As I shall demonstrate later, the myth and the phenomenon of vampirism and some allied states can only really be understood when certain metabolic, nutritional, and toxicological factors are taken into account. At some periods in history such factors may have served to compound and give concrete form to an underlying and emotionally pervasive mythology or cult in communities prone to superstition.

Although I shall endeavour to avoid sensationalism and an undue sense of the dramatic in this book, some of the cases and incidents to be reported achieved an inevitable degree of notoriety in their time. For this reason I must emphasise that I am dealing with *comparatively* rare instances of very bizarre conduct. I emphasise the word *comparatively*, because, for many years, I have been increasingly convinced that many more people engage in a range of strange activities than ever see the light of day, let alone the glare of media publicity. When such behaviours do come to light we have to try to suspend our disbelief and acknowledge that there is much about human behaviour that we simply do not understand. Neither the aetiological wisdom of psychiatry, nor the learning derived from anthropology, sociology, and theology can lay total claim to explanation. Suspension of disbelief, though extremely difficult, will lead, one hopes, to empathic understanding of some of the more bizarre conditions to be described in this book. This is its main purpose. Although there is a considerable literature on some of the topics presented, much of it is not easily accessible to busy practitioners or to the interested general reader.[6] Because of this, I hope that the work will be of interest to a variety of people who have professional involvement in this field. I have in mind psychiatrists, psychologists, social workers, general practitioners and physicians, nurses, penal staff, and those who, through the churches of various denominations, have a pastoral responsibility. I hope that it will also be useful to a group of people who often find themselves the front-line recipients of bizarre behaviours; I mean, of course, the police. Finally, I hope it will be of interest to the general reader who is genuinely fascinated by the wide diversity of behaviour shown by his or her fellows.[7]

The original impetus for the book grew out of my long-standing professional interest in people showing deviant behaviour (particularly those who had offended and were adjudged to be mentally disturbed); this found expression in two earlier works – *Offenders: Deviants or Patients?* (Tavistock 1980) and *Dangerous Behaviour: The Law and Mental Disorder* (Tavistock 1986). A few years ago this interest received further momentum as a result of a fairly modest attempt to explore the dual but highly related worlds of mythical and clinical vampirism.[8] The present offering represents a *narrowing* of my earlier focus to some extent; at the same time I hope that readers will be able to *broaden* the context of their own understanding from the more highly selected material to be presented here. In order to preserve the flow of the text, references within it have been kept to a minimum, but significant sources are referred to at the end of each chapter. The reader wishing to explore the topics further would do well to consult them. In some respects the notes and references may be considered more important than the text.

Notes and references

1. Detailed accounts of the so-called 'Hungerford massacre' can be found in the *Independent* for 20, 21, 22 August, 25, 26, 29, 30 September and 1 October 1987. The leading articles and letters in the issue for 21 August are also of interest.

2. The famous (or infamous) case of David Berkowitz ('The Son of Sam') is an interesting example. Berkowitz terrorised the citizens of New York during the period 1976–77, killing six people and wounding seven others. See T. Szasz, *Insanity, the Idea and its Consequences*, New York, Wiley, 1987, pp. 206–207. See also the account of the life and crimes of the serial killer Joseph Kallinger in F.R. Schreiber, *The Shoe Maker (The Anatomy of a Psychotic)*, Harmondsworth, Penguin Books, 1984. Other illustrations of large-scale and bizarre killings may be found in E. Revitch and L.B. Schlesinger, *Psychopathology of Homicide*, Illinois, Charles C. Thomas, 1981. The case of the mass killer Dennis Nilsen is discussed in Chapter five below.

3. Jung's writing is complex and his more metaphysical work is not easy to assimilate. One often feels that there must be some 'key' to the fund of knowledge that is locked in an illusive code. However, the effort to get to grips with the Jungian perspective is well worth while for those who wish to understand not only the importance of symbolism but the more illusive and troubling aspects of their fellow human beings' behaviour. A useful contemporary perspective may be found in A. Samuels, *Jung and the Post-Jungians*, London, Routledge and Kegan Paul, 1985.

4. See D. Goldstein, *Jewish Mythology*, Twickenham, Hamlyn, 1987. For a detailed exposition of the Tarot see A. Douglas, *The Tarot, the Origins, Meaning and Uses of the Cards*, Harmondsworth, Penguin Books, 1974.

5. See R.M. Bell, *Holy Anorexia*, Chicago, Chicago University Press, 1985. Of associated interest are the phenomena of stigmata – the reproduction through the ages of the wounds of Christ and similar signs. A number of the females showing such signs lived lives not unlike those of the early anorexics. Writing of stigmata, Wilson (1988) suggests that 'the whole phenomenon is undeniably bizarre, and yet the observations are too persistent and too consistent for it all to be dismissed as make-believe', I. Wilson, *The Bleeding Mind: An Investigation into the Mysterious Phenomenon of Stigmata*, London, Weidenfeld and Nicolson, 1988, p. 71.

6. There are very few easily accessible books on these topics. Two useful

exceptions are: C.T.H. Friedmann and R.A. Faguet (eds), *Extraordinary Disorders of Human Behaviour*, New York, Plenum Press, 1982, and M.D. Enoch and W.H. Trethowan, *Uncommon Psychiatric Syndromes* (2nd edn), Bristol, Wright and Sons, 1979.

7. For those unfamiliar with psychiatric signs and symptoms a recent work by Sims is strongly recommended: A. Sims, *Symptoms in the Mind: An Introduction to Descriptive Psychopathology*, London, Ballière Tindall, 1988.

8. See Chapter five below.

Chapter two

Some less familiar psychiatric conditions

'Be thou familiar, but by no means vulgar.'
(*Hamlet*, Act I, Scene iii)

The distinction between some of the conditions now to be described and those to be dealt with in the chapters that follow is somewhat arbitrary; it is provided mainly to facilitate presentation. Those described in this chapter would be regarded by common consent as psychiatric in the more conventional meaning of that term. But, as we shall see, those described in other chapters are, to some extent, less sharply delineated as psychiatric illnesses.

To the general reader, most psychiatric conditions must be less familiar since psychiatric disorders are, by definition, an indication of an apparent departure from normal. However, as a result of the popularisation of psychiatry many lay people will have some idea of what is meant by depression, mania, schizophrenia, and the various neuroses, even though their knowledge may be inaccurate to some degree.[1] In this chapter, certain infrequently seen conditions are described which are characterised by somewhat bizarre or unusual features. For this reason they might be said to represent the more extreme end of the psychiatric spectrum. However, having said this, it is as well to recall the caution expressed in Chapter one that behaviour that appears to be very bizarre and unusual may be but an extension of so-called normality. It is the *severity* and *intensity* of the condition that may set it apart. It is also important to remember that the prevalence of mental disturbances and the manner in which they are viewed appear to change at different periods of history.[2] In addition, there is considerable debate as to the aetiology (causes) of mental disorders. There are those who seek them in biological factors and those who see many, if not all, mental disorders as being explicable in terms of culture and environment. There are even those who suggest that mental disorders do not exist.[3] Those of more moderate views would suggest that, although many forms of mental disorder currently defy satisfactory explanation, it is probable that the truth is likely to lie somewhere between the two extreme perspectives referred to above, namely that a predisposition to mental disorder (however caused) is likely to make an individual more vulnerable to its manifestation if there are environmental stresses and/or precipitants. It is important to bear these caveats in mind in considering the selection of unusual psychiatric syndromes described below.

Some sinister and singular preoccupations

From time to time most of us have held strong and persistent feelings about others – for example, feelings of love, hate, or envy. Occasionally, such feelings may have led us to flout convention or even the law. For the most part, even though such feelings may lead people into difficulties they are usually held in check by the guidance and intervention of others, be they family, friends, or professional counsellors. However, for some people, the beliefs are so intrusive, irrational, and intense that no amount of normal persuasion will deflect the individual from holding to their convictions. Professional mental health workers often call such disorders of thinking 'monosymptomatic' because they occur in a singular and specific fashion and are not usually associated with any other disorder of thinking or behaviour. (A good illustration would be the delusional beliefs held by Peter Sutcliffe. He felt he had a mission to rid the world of prostitutes. Apart from this belief and its tragic outcome for all concerned, he appeared to be perfectly sane and rational in all other respects. It was mainly this that led to the controversy over the psychiatric evidence given at his trial.) This capacity to present as being perfectly sane and purposive is a snare for the lay person and the inexperienced professional worker. In their less florid presentations these beliefs are sometimes referred to as 'over-valued ideas' – abnormal beliefs which dominate the person's life.[4] Many of these disordered beliefs are also referred to as paranoid in nature; that is they are predominantly self-referrent. They may not, as is presupposed by common usage of the word, necessarily involve a singular and compelling degree of suspiciousness and feelings of persecution, though the first disorder to be described contains just these elements.[5]

Delusional jealousy

A degree of jealousy or envy is present in most people and it is only when shown to a pathological degree that mental health and other professionals are likely to become involved. Its manifestations will inevitably cover a wide spectrum. One sufferer has graphically described her intense jealousy towards her partner; this became so severe that it caused her to develop panic attacks and bouts of nausea. In her case, a long search for treatment succeeded; she found a therapist who engaged her in a form of therapy which helped her to establish the trigger factors that sparked off what, in her case, were neurotically and not psychotically based beliefs.[6] A more sinister and potentially highly dangerous variant of the disorder is that known as delusional, morbid, or sexual jealousy. (There appears to be some disagreement among psychiatrists as to the term preferred to describe the syndrome and the choice has varied thoughout this century.) The disorder has been known since earliest times and is well described in myth, legend, and literature. So graphically does Shakespeare depict the irrational nature of the condition in *Othello* that one variant of the disorder has become known as the 'Othello syndrome'.[7]

> 'O! beware, my lord, of jealousy;
> It is the green ey'ed monster which doth mock
> The meat it feeds on.'
> (*Othello*, Act III, Scene iii)

It is characterised by a central preoccupation with sexual infidelity. There is an unshakeable and irrational belief that the spouse or partner has been unfaithful. Innocent signs (for example, a light being switched on in a neighbour's house) are misinterpreted to mean that the person with whom the partner is having a relationship is signalling a time for an illicit meeting. As a result of the delusional beliefs the sufferer will follow the spouse or partner, keep them or have them kept under surveillance, and go to quite bizarre lengths to confirm their false beliefs. For example, by examining the spouse's or partner's underclothes for signs of seminal staining. There is no generally accepted explanation for the development of the disorder (which is usually found in males), but it has been suggested that the person suffering from the delusion may have behaved promiscuously in the past and have an expectation that the spouse or partner will behave in a similar fashion. Other explanations have suggested the possibility of impotence in the sufferer with consequent projection of a feeling of failure on to the spouse or partner. Another explanation stresses the possibility of repressed homosexuality resulting in phantasies about the spouse's or partner's male consort. It is not uncommon for the harassed and followed spouse or partner to admit the alleged infidelity in the hope that the hounding will then cease. Alas, this is not the case; such admission (seen by the sufferer from the delusion as a 'confession') may merely confirm them in their delusional beliefs and they may then cause serious injury or even death to the innocent victim of their delusions. The condition is regarded by most authorities as intractable. The nineteenth-century physician, Clouston, is quoted as saying:

> I now have in an asylum two quite rational-looking men, whose chief delusion is that their wives, both women of undoubted good character, have been unfaithful to them. Keep them off that subject and they are rational. But on that subject they are utterly delusional and insane.[8]

The quotation illustrates the circumscribed and encapsulated nature of the disordered thinking referred to earlier. Realistic (some might say cynical) observers of the condition have suggested that the most effective form of treatment may be geographical; that is, advise the spouse or partner to change her location and her name. Occasionally, when the individual suffering from such a delusion has been institutionalised for a delusionally inspired offence against the spouse or partner, it may be helpful to include a no-contact condition in their order for discharge if they are released under statutory supervision. At least this enables the possibility of recall to an institution to be considered in the event of declared intentions or actual manifestations of contact. The delusions are also seen in some organic states such as 'punch-drunkenness' and in cases of serious alcohol abuse. An associated disorder which may lead to a violent outcome is that of delusions of poisoning. In such cases sufferers may believe that close relatives and others near to them are attempting to poison them.[9]

Some other singular delusional states

There is a wide variety of other serious disorders of belief. There is the disorder known as erotomania, or *psychose passionnelle*, in which, customarily a woman (but not exclusively so),[10] believes that a man, usually older and socially quite unrealistically attainable (such as an important public figure) is in love with her. A variant of this disorder of thinking is known as de Clérambault's syndrome, after the French physician who first identified it. Such patients can cause a great deal of nuisance and embarrassment to those who are the object of their irrational and delusional beliefs. There is another group of related disorders in which the key characteristic is the belief that a person or persons close to the sufferer has or have been replaced by a double or doubles. Although these delusions have been described mainly in the psychiatric literature during this last century, the phenomena have existed for centuries in one form or another in folklore and legend. A similar phenomenon exists in the legendary accounts of 'changelings' left in place of another child. Readers will recall that in Shakespeare's *A Midsummer Night's Dream*, the quarrel between Titania and Oberon centres around the changeling child being brought up by Titania whom Oberon covets for his page. Such presentations are also not far removed from the numerous accounts in literary works of the *doppelgänger* phenomenon which is a purely subjective experience of doubling (as in Robert Louis Stevenson's *The Master of Ballantrae* and in Dostoevsky's *The Double*). Delusions of misidentification are seen in at least four closely related states:

1. the Capgras syndrome, in which the sufferer believes that an individual closely connected to him has been replaced by an exact replica;[11]
2. the syndrome of intermetamorphosis, in which the sufferer claims that the person close to him or her (and frequently regarded as a persecutor) and the incorrectly identified stranger share both physical and psychological similarities;
3. the syndrome of Frégoli, in which a false identification of persons closely connected with the sufferer occurs in strangers (the syndrome is named after a famous Italian actor and impersonator);
4. the syndrome of subjective doubles. Here, the sufferer believes that another individual has been transformed into his or her own self.

Recent accounts in the psychiatric literature suggest that the above syndromes and their variants may occur more frequently than was thought to have been the case in the past.[12] Other related and unusual delusional states that have been described in clinical practice include delusions of poverty and nihilism (Cotard's syndrome), severe hypochondriacal delusions (see also discussion of the Koro syndrome in Chapter four), and delusions of infestation (Ekbom's syndrome)[13] in which the sufferer believes he or she is infested. Communicated insanity, in which the delusions of one mentally ill individual are transferred to a significant other or others has also been described as have multiple (plusieurs) states such as *folie à trois* and *folie à quatre*.[14]

An addiction to hospitals

Most of us would find it hard to believe that there are people who persistently seek admission to hospital for self-induced complaints and in the process expose themselves to all manner of highly unpleasant investigations and surgical procedures. The person seeking such admission frequently gives highly plausible reasons for seeking it, fanciful accounts of their life histories (which are found subsequently to be quite untrue), and frequently take their discharge from hospital before medical and other investigations are completed. Although behaviour of this type has been known for centuries, it was not until the early 1950s that it was given the eponymous title of the *Munchausen* syndrome – after the famous eighteenth-century nobleman who was a great fabricator and wanderer. The appellation is not entirely apposite, because as far as one can tell from his chronicler, the good Baron was not addicted to hospital treatment and investigations for fictitious illnesses. In addition, he was, by all accounts, a far more attractive and congenial character than most of his modern counterparts.[15] A number of synonyms for the disorder have been proposed, but most have been discarded; for example, 'hospital hoboes', 'perigrinating problem patients', 'hospital addicts', and sufferers from 'factitious illness'. The key features of pathological lying (pseudologia fantastica) and self-induced physical symptomatology are usually accompanied by a very hostile, demanding, and unco-operative attitude. When confronted with their feigned signs and symptoms they become very angry and, as already noted, take their own discharge. A small number do not, and it may be that this latter group are the true hospital addicts described in the literature.[16] The presentation of the disorder can be very varied; and for this reason the term 'Munchausen syndrome' is considered by some to be a misnomer for a wide range of conditions whose central core is a disorder of the personality. It is obviously important to attempt to distinguish the condition from genuine cases of hysteria and from malingering (where the presentation of feigned signs and symptoms may serve some fraudulent purpose).[17] However, the borderlines are not always easy to establish.

The central characteristics of the condition appear to be: (1) satisfaction derived from manipulating the provisions of medical and surgical care; (2) satisfaction derived from exposure to recurring anaesthetic procedures (a stimulus akin maybe to 'dicing with death'); (3) receipt of highly personalised affection and warmth from medical and nursing staff (many of these patients come from unloving and highly disordered family backgrounds and live semi-nomadic and rootless lives); (4) stimulation derived from diagnostic and treatment procedures (akin perhaps to the need for continual excitement shown by some true psychopaths); (5) access to pain-killing agents (akin perhaps to some other forms of drug abuse); (6) provision of a safe, warm, haven within hospital (a search for 'asylum' in the original meaning of the word). Such a diverse assortment of possible motives would support the claim for multiple causation suggested in the clinical literature.[18] It follows, therefore, that the management of such 'patients' must be broadly based and take into account the fact that such long-standing patterns of behaviour are likely to prove highly unresponsive to most therapeutic endeavours. Some aspects of the condition, and the problems of differential diagnosis, are illustrated by the following two examples reported in the press. The first case involved court proceedings, though these are not a very common outcome of this kind of conduct.

A barman tricked 23 hospitals into giving him bed and breakfast – with the help of a small stone. [He] hid the stone under his back on hospital X-Ray tables to make it appear that he had a kidney stone. He admitted obtaining hospital services by deception ... 'I do it when I get somewhere and don't have the money to get bed and breakfast.' A psychiatrist told the court that 'the defendant suffered from an illness known as "hospital hopping" or Munchausen's syndrome.' The defendant was placed on probation with a requirement that he undertake psychiatric treatment.[19]

The second example comes from Holland and not only illustrates the wide range of symptoms encountered but, in addition, their connection with other disorders, in this case 'binge eating' (bulimia).

A woman made regular and persistent claims that she had taken overdoses of tranquillisers so that she could be stomach-pumped. However, after she was admitted to the Dutch National Poison Control Centre (where she was found to be atypically co-operative) her stomach, when emptied, was found to contain large quantities of recently digested food but no signs of drugs. It was discovered subsequently that she had been admitted to hospital in similar circumstances on at least 75 previous occasions, usually straight from a restaurant after a good meal. It was further reported that she managed to repeat the exercise twice in nearby hospitals in the ensuing few days.[20]

In recent years a further variant of the Munchausen condition has been described – 'Munchausen syndrome by proxy'.[21] In these fairly rare cases a mother may inflict a variety of injuries upon her child with the result that the child is hospitalised and may undergo extensive medical and surgical exploratory procedures, some of them involving considerable trauma. In one case study the mother had a long history of Munchausen-type hospital admissions herself and over the years her three children had presented with similar histories.[22] In all such cases there appears to be a thread of attention-seeking behaviour and the derivation of vicarious satisfaction from the attention given to the child. It is obviously important to try to establish differential diagnosis from that of suspected child abuse as we normally understand it. It has been suggested that many mothers are relieved when they have been found out. In one case where the children were able to remain within the family but under medical supervision, the mother wrote to the physician 'I will forever thank God and you.'[23] One further example of a Munchausen-type condition is that of feigned bereavement. In this disorder significant facts are feigned or distorted in order to gain sympathy.[24]

Talking besides the point

The factitious qualities shown in Munchausen-type disorders highlight and enable us to examine briefly another somewhat similar and rare psychiatric presentation – the Ganser syndrome. In this condition we are not concerned as much with attempts to gain sympathy and attention as with *apparent* falsifications that seem to be designed to relieve the subject from an unpleasant or highly problematic situation. The disorder derives its name from the German physician, Ganser, who, in 1897, appears to have been the first medical man to have described the condition in any detail. However, some characteristics of the condition had been described in considerably earlier accounts.[25] In a public lecture which (in view of subsequent controversies as to the correct classification of the syndrome) Ganser interestingly entitled 'A peculiar hysterical state', he described a small number of patients who exhibited a cluster of somewhat unusual features which he suggested justified their being classed as a unique syndrome.

> The most obvious sign which they present consists of their inability to answer correctly the simplest questions which are asked of them, even though by many of their answers they indicate that they have grasped, in a large part, the sense of the question, and in their answers they betray at once a baffling ignorance and a surprising lack of knowledge which they assuredly once possessed or still possess.[26]

The above passage contains most of the essential features of this strange condition, notably the tendency to give approximate (and silly) answers and 'talking besides the point' (*vorbeigehen/*

vorbeireden). There is a considerable degree of disagreement in the clinical accounts as to the necessary presence of other features; indeed, there are those who consider that the condition is merely a variant of hysteria or even a conscious contrivance as in malingering. In order to make a substantive diagnosis of a true Ganser state it has been suggested that, in addition to the features already described, there should also be hallucinations, defects of memory, clouding of consciousness to varying degree, and subsequent and sudden complete recovery with amnesia for the whole episode.[27] For practical purposes it may be very difficult to distinguish a Ganser state from behaviour that can be attributable to a clear psychiatric illness, organic disorder, or, as already suggested, conscious simulation.[28] Ganser's original sample of cases consisted of prisoners and a number of later accounts have described individuals who had been institutionalised for a variety of reasons. However, it has also been seen in a variety of other settings. From a forensic-psychiatric point of view it has been well observed that its

> manifestly slight relationship with crime is probably dependent in the case of the symptom on the vigilance of prison medical officers in discouraging simulation, and in the case of the syndrome, on the similarly light correlation of crime with frank mental illness, *which is all the more reason for treating it with respect when it does appear*.[29] (Italics added.)

The disorder usually runs a natural course with a tendency towards eventual recovery. If the disorder is associated with an underlying psychotic illness (such as severe depression) appropriate treatment for the latter will be necessary. There is, therefore, good reason for hospitalising such patients so that detailed assessment may take place under the best possible conditions with a view to establishing pointers to correct diagnosis and subsequent treatment.[30]

Speaking with several voices

Disorders of personality have had a unique and controversial place in the history of psychiatry; for over a hundred years their phenomena, course, classification, and management have exercised the minds of a variety of disciplines claiming to have a valid interest in the subject. Contributions to the debate have come from psychiatrists and psychologists, but some of the more controversial have come from social scientists and lawyers who have raised important ethical and epistemological issues.[31]

It is not unreasonable to suggest that the personality disorders are the Achilles' heel of psychiatry. Numerous psychiatrists have often felt beleaguered when asked to justify the existence of the disorder in a court of law; many are somewhat reluctant to treat persons diagnosed as suffering from this group of conditions because they are not very rewarding patients. This is not the place to offer an extended treatment of personality disorder, but a few general observations may be helpful in providing a context for the more specific discussion of multiple personality disorder to follow.[32] Many authorities have drawn attention to the complexities involved in trying to establish a conceptual framework for an understanding of *temperament, personality*, and *personality disorder*. Rutter[33] has suggested that temperament is best defined in terms of simple, non-motivational, non-cognitive, stylistic characteristics that suggest meaningful ways of describing individual differences between people. These might be regarded as the soft 'data base' in terms of being less precise than personality, which differs from temperament in the sense that the former includes the integrative, organisational, and motivational elements, among others. Although personality disorder is an illusive concept, three underlying essential features can be discerned: (1) an onset in childhood or adolescence; (2) a long-standing persistence over time without any substantial remission; (3) abnormalities that seem to represent a basic aspect of the individual's usual functioning. Shakespeare's depiction of the early character and development of Richard III – as seen through the eyes of his mother – the aged Duchess of York – gives the essential 'feel' of the condition.

> 'Thou cam'st on earth to make the earth my hell.
> A grievous burden was thy birth to me;
> Tetchy and wayward was thy infancy;
> Thy school-days frightful, desp'rate, wild and furious.
> Thy prime of manhood daring, bold and venturous;
> Thy age confirmed, proud, subtle and bloody,
> More mild but yet more harmful, kind in hatred:
> What comfortable hour canst thou name
> That ever graced me in thy company?'
> (*Richard III*, Act IV, Scene iv)

The last hundred years have witnessed various trends in approaches to the study of personality disorders; the traditional psychiatric; the postulation of some psychological defect; the social deviancy approach; the psychodynamic and the psychoanalytic; and, in more recent years, neuro-psycho-physiological approaches.[34] It is hardly surprising, in view of the shadowy nature of the concept, that no single approach has met with universal acceptance. However, despite divergencies of opinion as to aetiology and classification, follow-up studies tend to suggest that an overall diagnosis of personality disorder has satisfactory reliability and reasonable predictive validity.[35]

It has been suggested that two broad groupings of personality disorders may be discerned currently. The first includes several categories that can be more appropriately grouped as variants of disorders such as affective disorder, autism, and schizophrenia. The second grouping consists of disorders characterised by a persistent abnormality in general social functioning – as, for example, in severe psychopathic disorder.[36] The sub-group now to be considered – *multiple personality disorder* – has some highly unusual characteristics. Interest in dual and multiple personality is not new; there are a number of illustrations in literature of dual personality, for example, Hoffman's *The Devil's Elixir*, first published in this country in 1824 and James Hogg's famous account in his *Memoirs and Confessions of a Justified Sinner*, published in the same year.[37] The concept has always aroused considerable interest, not least among the media, and some of the more sensational cases have eventually found their way into television and/or film. One of the earliest clinical accounts appears to be that by Mitchill;[38] subsequent depictions had been provided by Morton Prince, Thigpen and Cleckley and much more recently by the non-medical observer, Schreiber.[39] Recent studies by a variety of workers indicate that the disorder may not be quite as rare as some of the earlier writers on the topic thought. However, it has also been suggested that the medical attention such persons receive may merely serve to facilitate the expression of the symptomatology and add to its proliferation.[40] This is one reason for thinking that the disorder may have become more 'fashionable' in recent years. The picture is complicated further by the fact that the presentation of the disorder may occasionally be masked by other symptoms, thus making the validity of the disorder as a discrete entity somewhat questionable. An added difficulty is that multiple personality disordered patients have a tendency towards secretiveness. The most up-to-date and generally accepted diagnostic criteria are:

A. The existence within the person of two or more distinct personalities or personality states (each with its own relatively enduring pattern of perceiving, relating to, and thinking about the environment and self).
B. At least two of these personalities or personality states recurrently [taking] full control of the person's behaviour.[41]

The presentation is likely to be characterised by the on-going co-existence of relatively consistent, but alternate, separate, sometimes *very numerous* identities with recurring episodes of distortion of memory and frank amnesia. It is the recurrence and co-existence of these multiple presentations that give the disorder its bizarre quality. The individual may also exhibit hallucinations, formal symptoms of schizophrenia, and in some cases depressive symptomatology. Certain essential features may be summarised: (1) amnesic periods, subjectively and objectively observed; (2) abuse in childhood, particularly of a serious nature (for example, coercive incestuous relationships); (3) a stormy psychiatric history with hysterical features. The condition has been explained in psychodynamic terms as making use of the unconscious mechanism of dissociation as a defence, allowing complete repression of unacceptable memories for an earlier period. Subsequently, the whole personality may return from repression and 'take over' as an alternative personality or personalities. Sufferers tend to be of superior intelligence, though this is by no means universal. They may present occasionally as suffering from 'black-outs' and they frequently have long histories of therapy of one kind or another. A history of alcohol, other drug abuse, and suicide attempts is not uncommon. Because multiple personality disorder presents in such a multi-faceted fashion and its aetiology is uncertain, treatment approaches have to be based upon sound differential diagnosis and an eclectic approach. In some cases hypnotherapy has been found to be a useful therapeutic adjunct; a number of patients seem to recognise that something is amiss, but that they require help over a long period. Children seem to be particularly susceptible to treatment. Differential diagnosis can be aided by careful scrutiny for the existence of a number of the following indicators: (1) previous failure in treatment; (2) three or more previous diagnoses of mental illness; (3) severe headaches that have proved to be resistant to medication; (4) presence of current psychiatric *and somatic symptoms*; (5) a history of time distortion or time lapses; (6) the patient having been informed of behaviour that he or she has not remembered; (7) the patient having been informed of observed changes in his or her face, voice, and behavioural style; (8) discovery by the patient of possessions, products, or 'alien' handwriting that he or she cannot recognise or account for; (9) recurrence of auditory hallucinations (which in view of the problems of differential diagnosis, referred to earlier, require special care in assessment); (10) a history of child abuse, particularly of a serious or sadistic nature (see earlier comments, above); (11) the patient's use of the word 'we' in a collective sense.[42]

Finally, the elicitation of what appear to be separate personalities with hypnosis or hypnotic drugs may suggest, but not necessarily confirm, the disorder. Great caution needs to be exercised in interpreting the results of such endeavours. It may be all too easy for the therapist unconsciously to perpetuate the symptoms in a collusive relationship with this particular type of patient. Although his remarks were made in the last century, one is still mindful of Axel Munthe's reservations about Charcot's famous demonstrations of so-called hypnosis at La Salpêtrière.[43]

Conclusion

This chapter has been concerned with a brief review of some unusual disorders of human behaviour which seem to lie reasonably clearly within the psychiatric domain. However, it will have been readily observed that there is not only considerable debate as to how such disorders should be classified, but that uncertainty exists about treatment and prognosis. In the following chapters we shall be concerned with behaviours that appear to stand more at the boundaries of psychiatry and which demonstrate the relevance of cultural perspective and diversity. Finally, it is important to stress once again the degree of selectivity exercised in the presentation of all these states.

Notes and references

1. For a useful and highly readable survey of the main psychiatric disorders, their likely causes, classification, and treatment see A. Clare, *Psychiatry in Dissent: Controversial Issues in Thought and Practice* (2nd edn), London, Tavistock, 1980 (particularly Chapters 1 and 2).
2. See Chapter one above and H. Prins, 'Understanding Insanity: Some Glimpses into Historical Fact and Fiction', *British Journal of Social Work*, 1987, vol. 17, pp. 91–98.
3. See, for example, T. Szasz, *Insanity, the Idea and Its Consequences*, New York, Wiley, 1987. For a spirited refutation of his views see M. Roth and J. Kroll, *The Reality of Mental Illness*, Cambridge, Cambridge University Press, 1986.
4. McKenna describes them as 'a solitary, abnormal (belief) that is neither delusional nor obsessional in nature, but which is preoccupying to the extent of dominating the sufferer's life', P.J. McKenna, 'Disorders with Over-valued Ideas', *British Journal of Psychiatry*, 1984, vol. 145, pp. 579–585.
5. The current edition of the *Diagnostic and Statistical Manual of Mental Disorders* (3rd edn revised), *DSM III(R)*, American Psychiatric Association, New York, 1987, uses the broad classification of delusional disorder (297:10, pp. 202–203). Within this classification several subtypes are specified; for example, erotomanic, grandiose, jealous, persecutory, somatic, and unspecified. See also A. Sims, *Symptoms of the Mind: An Introduction to Descriptive Psychopathology*,

London, Baillire Tindall, 1988, Chapter 7 and A. Munro, 'Paranoia Revisited', *British Journal of Psychiatry*, 1982, vol. 141, pp. 344–349, and A. Munro, 'Mono-symptomatic Hypochondriacal Psychosis', in K.J.B. Rix and R.P. Snaith (eds) *The Psychopathology of Body Image, British Journal of Psychiatry Supplement No. 2*, 1988, vol. 153, pp. 37–40 (*Proceedings of the Second Leeds Psychopathology Symposium*, 18–19 September 1986).

6. C. Aziz, 'Prey to the Green-Eyed Monster', *Independent*, 10 November 1987.

7. See M.D. Enoch, 'Sexual Jealousy', *British Journal of Sexual Medicine*, 1980, vol. 80, pp. 30–34 and M.D. Enoch and W.H. Trethowan, *Uncommon Psychiatric Syndromes* (2nd edn.), Bristol, Wright and Sons, 1979. The broad context of the disorder has been reviewed more recently by P.E. Mullen and L.H. Maack, 'Jealousy, Pathological Jealousy and Aggression', in D.P. Farrington and J. Gunn (eds), *Aggression and Dangerousness*, Chichester, Wiley, 1985.

8. Quoted in Enoch and Trethowan, op. cit. 1979, p. 47.

9. See D. Mawson, 'Delusions of Poisoning', *Medicine, Science and the Law*, 1985, vol. 25, pp. 279–287. See also K.W. de Pauw and T.K. Szulecka, 'Dangerous Delusions and the Misidentification Syndrome', *British Journal of Psychiatry*, 1988, vol. 152, pp. 91–96.

10. See P. Taylor, B. Mahendra and J. Gunn, 'Erotomania in Males', *Psychological Medicine*, 1983, vol. 13, pp. 645–650. The extent to which the so-called de Clérambault's syndrome should be described as a separate entity has recently been questioned. See P. Ellis and G. Mellsopp, 'De Clérambault's Syndrome – A Nosological Entity?', *British Journal of Psychiatry*, 1985, vol. 146, pp. 90–95. See also more generally F.D. Rudnick, 'The Paranoid-Erotic Syndromes', in C.T.H. Friedmann and R.H. Faguet (eds), *Extraordinary Disorders of Human Behaviour*, New York, Plenum Press, 1982, Chapter 7.

11. It has been recently suggested that the focus of the delusions in Capgras states can also apply to inanimate objects. See D.M. Anderson, 'The Delusion of Inanimate Doubles: Implications for Understanding the Capgras Phenomenon', *British Journal of Psychiatry*, 1988, vol. 153, pp. 694–699.

12. For a more extended treatment see Sims, op. cit. 1988, Chapter 7.

13. T.M. Reilly, 'Delusional Infestation', in K.J.B. Rix and R.P. Snaith, op. cit. 1988, pp. 44–46.

14. A. Sims, P. Solomons and P. Humphreys, 'Folie à Quatre', *British Journal of Psychiatry*, 1977, vol. 130, pp. 134–138.

15. Further details of the historical aspects of this disorder and its presentation may be found in Enoch and Trethowan, op. cit. 1979, Chapter 6 and in C.V. Ford, 'Munchausen Syndrome', in Friedmann and Faguet, op. cit. 1982, Chapter 2.

16. For an attempt at differential diagnosis see L. Cheng and L. Hummell, 'The Munchausen Syndrome as a Psychiatric Condition', *British Journal of Psychiatry*, 1978, vol. 133, pp. 20–21. For further amplification of this aspect and varieties of presentation see also

B. Blackwell, 'The Munchausen Syndrome', in T. Silverstone and B. Barraclough (eds), *Contemporary Psychiatry*, Ashford, Kent, Headley Bros., 1975, pp. 391–398. See also G.G. Hay, 'Feigned Psychosis: A Review of the Simulation of Mental Illness', *British Journal of Psychiatry*, 1983, vol. 143, pp. 8–10; T. Wimberley, 'The Making of a Munchausen', *British Journal of Medical Psychology*, 1981, vol. 54, pp. 121–129; M.W.P. Carney and J.P. Brown, 'Clinical Features and Motives among 42 Artefactual Illness Patients', *British Journal of Medical Psychology*, 1983, vol. 56, pp. 57–66. A mythological and cultural context is provided by A. Cremona-Barbaro, 'Munchausen Syndrome and its Symbolic Significance', *British Journal of Psychiatry*, 1987, vol. 151, pp. 76–79.

17. A. Sims, op. cit. 1988, pp. 182–184.
18. A. Sims, ibid.
19. *Independent*, 8 August 1987. Because of the time taken up by these patients in busy hospital departments and because it is difficult to keep track of them, it has been suggested that professional organisations such as the Royal College of Psychiatrists might institute a central register of such cases. See A. Markantonakis and A.S. Lee, 'Psychiatric Munchausen's Syndrome: A College Register?', Letter, *British Journal of Psychiatry*, 1988, vol. 153, p. 403. There is some evidence to suggest that the *psychiatric presentation* of the syndrome may be increasing. See M.E. Jones and M.P. Sternberg, 'Munchausen's Syndrome', *British Journal of Psychiatry*, 1985, vol. 147, pp. 729–730.
20. *Independent*, 14 June 1988.
21. R. Meadow, 'Munchausen Syndrome by Proxy: The Hinterland of Child-abuse', *Lancet*, 1977, vol. ii, pp. 343–345. See also A. Spackman, 'Parents who Secretly Injure a Child', *Independent*, 1 December 1987.
22. See D. Black, 'The Extended Munchausen Syndrome: A Family Case', *British Journal of Psychiatry*, 1981, vol. 138, pp. 466–469.
23. Spackman, op. cit., p. 13.
24. J. Snowden, R. Solomons and M. Druce, 'Feigned Bereavement – Twelve Cases', *British Journal of Psychiatry*, 1978, vol. 133, pp. 15–19.
25. See Enoch and Trethowan, op. cit. 1979, pp. 51–52.
26. This passage is a translation by C.E. Schorer of Ganser's original paper. See C.E. Schorer, 'The Ganser Syndrome', *British Journal of Criminology*, 1965, vol. 5, pp. 120–131.
27. Enoch and Trethowan, op. cit. 1979.
28. Enoch and Trethowan, ibid.
29. P.D. Scott, 'Commentary' on Schorer's paper, *British Journal of Criminology*, 1965, vol. 5, pp. 127–134. See also D.B. Auerbach, 'The Ganser Syndrome', in Friedmann and Faguet, op. cit. 1982, Chapter 3.
30. See R. Latcham, A. White and A. Sims, 'Ganser Syndrome: The Aetiological Argument', *Journal of Neurology, Neurosurgery and Psychiatry*, 1978, vol. 41, pp. 851–854. See also M.W.P. Carney, T.K.N. Chary, P. Robotis and A. Childs, 'Ganser Syndrome and its

Management', *British Journal of Psychiatry*, 1987, vol. 151, pp. 697–700. An unusual case of its presentation in a child is to be found in P.D. Dabhalkar, 'Ganser Syndrome: A Case Report and Discussion', *British Journal of Psychiatry*, 1987, vol. 151, pp. 256–258.

31. See, for example, B. Wootton, *Social Science and Social Pathology*, London, Allen and Unwin, 1959, pp. 256–258.
32. See H. Prins, 'The Status of Personality Disorder', *Current Opinion in Psychiatry*, 1988, vol. 1, pp. 184–187.
33. M. Rutter, 'Temperament, Personality and Personality Disorder', *British Journal of Psychiatry*, 1987, vol. 150, pp. 443–458.
34. M. Rutter, op. cit. 1987.
35. M. Rutter, op. cit. 1987.
36. For a summary of views on psychopathic personality disorder see H. Prins, *Dangerous Behaviour: The Law and Mental Disorder*, London, Tavistock, 1986, Chapter 5.
37. On some aspects of the origins of the concept of dual personality see B. Clarke, 'Arthur Wigan and the Duality of Mind', *Psychological Medicine*, Monographs, Supplement No. 11, Cambridge, Cambridge University Press, 1987, pp. 25–42.
38. S.L. Mitchill, 'A Double Consciousness, or a Duality of Person in the Same Individual', *Medical Repository*, 1816, vol. 3, pp. 185–186. Quoted in T.A. Fahy, 'The Diagnosis of Multiple Personality Disorder: A Critical Review', *British Journal of Psychiatry*, 1988, vol. 153, pp. 597–606.
39. M. Prince, *The Dissociation of Personality*, New York, Longman, 1905; C.H. Thigpen and H. Cleckley, *The Three Faces of Eve*, London, Secker and Warburg, 1957; F.R. Schreiber, *Sybil*, New York, Regnery Books, 1973.
40. See Sims, op. cit. 1988, pp. 154–155 and Fahy, op. cit. 1988, p. 604. See also T.A. Fahy, M. Abas and J.C. Brown, 'Multiple Personality: A Symptom of Psychiatric Disorder', *British Journal of Psychiatry*, 1989, vol. 154, pp. 99–101.
41. American Psychiatric Association, *Diagnostic and Statistical Manual of Mental Disorders* (3rd edn revised), *DSM II(R)*, 1987, p. 272.
42. I have drawn here upon a useful and comprehensive survey by R.P. Kluft, 'An Update on Multiple Personality Disorder', *Hospital and Community Psychiatry*, 1987, vol. 38, pp. 363–373.
43. A. Munthe, *The Story of San Michele*, London, John Murray, 1949, Chapters 18 and 19. See also Fahy, op. cit. 1988, p. 604.

Chapter three

Besieged by devils: possession and possession states

'Beware you do not conjure up a spirit you cannot lay.'
(Ben Johnson, *The New Inn*, Act III, Scene ii)

'Farewell the tranquil mind: farewell content.'
(*Othello*, Act III, Scene iii)

Background and perspective

The phenomenon of an alien presence or spirit entering and taking control of an individual is as old as civilisation itself. As we shall see, numerous explanations have been put forward; in the final analysis we may have to suspend our disbelief in those cases where rational and medical explanations seem to fail us. Historical, biblical, archaeological, and contemporary evidence indicates its presence in diverse forms and in all cultures; for example, in Babylonia, in Ethiopia, Nigeria, Greece, Tibet, Haiti, and throughout Europe. Primitive cave drawings, such as those found at Trois Frères in France, support early historical accounts of outbreaks of ecstatic and trance-like dancing, such as those depicted in thirteenth-century Italy as the 'dancing mania'. It has been well stated that 'the phenomenon of "spirit communication" in mediumistic trance, of "spirit possession" and of "demonopathy" are closely related, and are known to both east and west ... these conditions ... present themselves in many countries and it is misconceived to think that they are to be found only in outlandish cultures'.[1] Possession is an emotive word; some prefer the term *oppression* or *obsession*, but to me these do not appear to convey the full force of what is best regarded as the alien experience implied in the word possession. The words demonic *influence* are sometimes used for the more mild forms of the phenomena and demonic *oppression* for the more serious; demonic *attack* for their more acute manifestation.[2] The word *obsession* is often taken to describe a psychological concept in which the victim's mind remains his or her own, whereas in *possession*, the victim's mind is taken over altogether and held to be occupied by some malevolent force.[3] Some credibility seems to be given to this view when we consider that people wishing to disclaim responsibility for an act often say 'I don't know what possessed me.' Some people see in possession states an attempt to disclaim responsibility for actions that would normally be disapproved of, or punished by, society – for example, uttering obscenities or engaging in coercive sexual practices. It is also of interest to note in passing that in ancient times victims of possession were sometimes referred to as 'energumen' – from the Greek word 'ergon' meaning work. This word encapsulated the belief that the devil was thought to work within them.[4]

There is an additional perspective to be considered by way of introduction. This concerns the framework within which societies seek scapegoats and explanations for phenomena they do not readily understand. Non-comprehension breeds fear, and fear readily produces severe and repressive measures. For example, the more gentle commands of Jesus to evil spirits to depart were not always echoed in practice by those who came after Him. Those said to be possessed by demons, or who were considered to be witches, were subjected to various forms of much less gentle exorcism such as torture and mutilation before they were put to death in barbaric fashion. In very early times, the technique of trephining (making small holes in the skull) was used to allow evil spirits to escape. In later times, as well as various forms of torture, such measures as enemas and emetics were used. In the latter part of the Middle Ages one of the most influential manuals for the examination of those thought to be possessed and to be indulging in the practice of witchcraft was the infamous *Malleus Malleficarum* or *Witches' Hammer*, written by two Dominican inquisitors, James Sprenger and Henry Kramer.[5] Various theories have been put forward to explain the very high proportion of women amongst those thought to be witches and those thought to be possessed. It has been suggested by one authority that 'women's possession cults are ... I argue thinly disguised movements against the dominant sex'.[6] The long-held view that all those thought to have been possessed in earlier times were suffering from some form of mental disorder has been challenged recently by those interested in psychiatric historiography. Examination of mediaeval and later sources suggests only a very limited connection between the two phenomena.[7] One writer has summed up the whole problem very succinctly in stating that 'Problems relating to mental health appear to be intrinsic to the nature of man and to reflect the impossibility of separating biological, psychological and cultural influences.'[8] Historical evidence also suggests that possession phenomena occur in periods of great social change and upheaval. It is worthy of note that in this country, from the 1970s onwards, there has been a considerable development of interest in occult practices and their depiction in the media – practices that have caused much disquiet among many people. Recent newspaper accounts have stressed the vulnerability of children and young people to occult experience and have outlined several case histories in support of the contention that black magic and occult practice are far more widespread than most people suppose. One mother has described how her 15-year-old son suddenly changed as a result of such 'dabbling'.

> One moment she thought she had a healthy rebellious teenager on her hands, the next, she was thrown into the world of the occult .... 'Sam [her son] suddenly burst in. We didn't recognise him. His whole face and body changed. He was spitting and speaking in a voice we hadn't heard before. He said he was a demon and was going to kill the family. Then he grabbed a knife from the kitchen drawer and went for my other son.'[9]

In the same article cases are cited in which children had been subjected to sexual abuse during occult sessions. The situation is considered to be so serious by some people that an organisation known as *The Reachout Trust* has been established to help those who are troubled by, and wish to sever their connections with, the occult. Such contemporary illustrations serve to reinforce the earlier statement that possession and allied disorders are neither the prerogative of so-called primitive cultures nor are they phenomena rooted solely in the past. As recently as August 1986, the Pope expressed his real fears about the power of the Devil as an angel who had rebelled against God.[10]

Some biblical allusions

Most people are reasonably familiar with some of the illustrations of demonic possession in the Bible, particularly those in the New Testament. They may be less familiar with some of the allusions to possession by evil spirits in the Old Testament. A good example of the latter is that of the troubled mind of King Saul. In the first *Book of Samuel* (19: 9 and 10) we find the words:

> An evil spirit from the Lord came upon Saul as he was sitting in the house with his spear in his hand; and David was playing the harp. Saul tried to pin David to the wall with the spear, but he avoided the King's thrust so that Saul drove the spear into the

wall. David escaped and got safely away.[11]

The account of the behaviour of the Babylonian King Nebuchadnezzar, when he felt he was being changed into a frightening animal, seems to be an early description of the Windigo phenomenon (see pp. 30 and 58): 'He was banished from the society of men and ate grass like oxen: his body was drenched by the dew of heaven, until his hair grew long like goats' hair and his nails like eagles' talons.' (*Book of Daniel* 4: 33; see also the discussion of lycanthropy in Chapter five.)

It seems quite clear that the notion of possession by an evil spirit was known and described in early Jewish history. It is certainly not a phenomenon making its first appearance in the Christian era. Some illustrations from the New Testament now follow and these provide a useful backcloth to the discussion that follows. In *Mark* 9: 20–27, we find a description of how Jesus was called to deal with the case of a boy who was thought to be possessed.

> 'Master, I brought my son to you. He is possessed by a spirit which makes him speechless. Whenever it attacks him, it dashes him to the ground, and he foams at the mouth, grinds his teeth, and goes rigid.'
> Jesus commanded the boy to be brought before him and having made careful enquiry of the boy's father as to the history of the boy's affliction proceeded to rebuke the unclean spirit in the following terms. 'Deaf and dumb spirit ... I command you, come out of him and never come back.' After crying aloud and racking him fiercely, it came out; and the boy looked like a corpse; in fact many said, 'He is dead.' But Jesus took his hand and raised him to his feet, and he stood up.

This extract is of considerable interest for three reasons. First, one interpretation of the boy's condition might have been that of an epileptiform illness (see pp. 29 and 33); second, the way in which Jesus took a careful 'history' from the father is an excellent example of what is required from anyone looking into a so-called possession state; third, it also illustrates the form of words that are sometimes used in exorcism ceremonies.

In *Mark* 1: 23 ff. we find the following passage:

> Now there was a man in the synagogue possessed by an unclean spirit. Jesus rebuked the spirit within the man and said 'Be silent and come out of him,' and the unclean spirit threw the man into convulsions and with a loud cry left him.

In *Mark* 1: 32–34, we also read the statement that at a large gather-
ing Jesus 'cast out devils' from a significant number of people. In
Luke 4: 1–13, there are a number of illustrations of the Devil attempting to enter Jesus and to possess Him. In *Matthew* 15: 21–28,
He is approached by a woman whose daughter is possessed of a devil.
He adjures her to be of good faith and the devil departs from her. In
the *Acts of the Apostles*, Paul is credited with acts of exorcism over
evil spirits (16: 16–18 and 19: 11–12). He achieves these in contrast
to 'unbelievers' who try to use exorcism by merely using the name of
Jesus (19: 13–20). The *manner* in which these spirits are ordered to
depart has already been commented upon; I shall return subsequently to the question of the beliefs and attitudes of those who
offer such a ministry of healing. Two further illustrations complete
this brief survey of possession phenomena in ancient times. The first
is from the fourth century AD and provides a very clear picture of the
main features of such states.

> The unclean devil, when he comes upon the soul of a man ...
> comes like a wolf upon a sheep, ravening for blood and ready to
> devour. His presence is most cruel; the sense of it most
> oppressive; the mind is darkened; his attack is an injustice also,
> and the usurpation of another's possession. For he tyrannically
> uses another's body, another's instruments, as his own property;
> he throws down him who stands upright ... he perverts the
> tongue and distorts the lips. Foam comes instead of words; the
> man is filled with darkness; his eye is open yet his soul sees not
> through it.[12]

The second is a sharply evocative illustration from roughly the same
period:

> But as soon as we enter the field of the divine combat (exorcism)
> and drive them forth with the arrow of the holy name of Jesus,
> then thou mayest take pity on the other – when thou shall have
> learned to know him – for that he is delivered over to such a
> fight. His face is suddenly deprived of colour, his body rises up
> of itself, the eyes in madness roll in their sockets and squint
> horribly, the teeth, covered with a horrible foam, grind between
> blue-white lips; and limbs twisted in all directions are given over
> to trembling; he sighs, he weeps; he fears the appointed day of
> Judgement and complains that he is driven out; he confesses his
> sex, the time and place he entered into the man.[13]

Some later illustrations

One of the best illustrations of 'mass' possession phenomena is to be found in the well-documented mid-seventeenth century case of the Ursuline nuns of Loudon. This story has been retold by a number of modern writers, including Aldous Huxley (*The Devils of Loudon*) and John Whiting (*The Devils*). One of the nuns was alleged to have been possessed by the demon Asmodeus:

> Asmodeus was not long in manifesting his supreme rage,
> shaking the girl backwards and forwards a number of times and
> making her strike like a hammer with such rapidity that her
> teeth rattled and sounds were forced out of her throat ...
> between these movements her face became completely
> unrecognisable, her glance furious, her tongue prodigiously
> large, long, and hanging down out of her mouth, livid and dry.[14]

In an eighteenth-century illustration, a pastor is trying to expel Satan from a woman deemed to be possessed. He had the woman brought into church and read from the Bible, while, according to the account, Satan scoffed at him through the mouth of the possessed woman.

> Satan broke into complaints against me: 'How dost thou
> oppress, how dost thou torment me ... ?' when at last I addressed
> to him the most violent exhortations in the name of Jesus, he
> cried out, 'Oh, I burn, I burn! Oh, what torture, what torture!',
> or loaded me with furious invectives ... During all these prayers,
> clamourings and disputes, Satan tortured the poor creature
> horribly, howled through her mouth in a frightful manner and
> threw her to the ground so rigid, so insensible that she became
> as cold as ice and lay as dead, at which time we could not
> perceive the slightest breath until, at last, with God's help she
> came to herself.[15]

Finally, a short nineteenth-century illustration. This concerned a boy of 10 who showed signs of possession when in the presence of churches or church regalia and ritual.

> ... the possessed uttered a terrible cry. We seemed no longer to
> hear a human voice but that of a savage animal ... we exposed
> the fragment of the Holy Cross. When the Sign of the Cross was
> made with it, the young man uttered an appalling scream. All
> the time he did not cease to spit forth vile insults against the
> fragment of the Cross and the two officiants [Father Regimus

and Father Aurelian] ... the clamour and the spitting lasted without interruption until the recitation of the litanies of the saints.[16]

As indicated earlier, it would be possible to try to explain many of the above phenomena in medical and psychiatric terms. Some psychiatrists, such as the late William Sargent (who became interested in the phenomena as a result of treating battle-induced neuroses in World War II) would emphasise an epileptic-type basis for some of the biblical and later illustrations.[17] It is perhaps not without significance that, for many centuries, epilepsy was known as the 'sacred disease', giving its sufferers at one and the same time a cachet of God-given power and a feared affliction. Psychiatrists with a less neurological orientation, as we shall see shortly, would proffer explanations in terms of hysterical manifestations in persons already vulnerable to the development of such conditions. Such individuals behave in a state known as hysterical dissociation in which, at the relevant time, they may not be aware of their own behaviour and attitudes. The history of psychiatry shows the power of suggestion and its effects upon vulnerable subjects – as evidenced in the work of both Mesmer and Charcot in the nineteenth century. Children may be particularly susceptible to suggestion. Some authorities have pointed to the suggestibility of both those 'observing' and those 'healing' individuals thought to be possessed. Though some medical authorities may be sceptical and highly critical of descriptions of such states as demonic possession, others believe that religion and prayer and their restorative forces have much to offer. One psychiatrist has described the case of a 13-year-old Yakima Indian girl living on a reservation in Central Washington State. She was referred to him with possession-like symptoms, but was only 'cured' after a form of ritual exorcism had taken place. In this case, the author thought that the girl and her family were torn between the demands of two cultures; because of this they needed the approaches of both modern psychiatry and more 'primitive' forms of healing. He also made the interesting (and not often noted) point that, once 'cured', victims may be thought to be invested henceforth with special powers.[18] An even more important point is worth making. In modern societies, where people of many beliefs and cultures now live alongside one another, it is vital to understand the context of these diverse beliefs in order to comprehend behaviour that may all too easily be given a psychiatric label. One final point can usefully be made at this stage. Some who regularly engage in trying to deal with the types of states described above may, over time, come to feel alienated or contaminated themselves, as did Father Surin, one of the priests who attempted to exorcise the Loudon nuns. He developed what appears to have been a severe depressive illness which lasted for more than twenty years. As we shall see, support of colleagues and of others is vital in dealing with these phenomena.

A brief cross-cultural perspective

In many cultures, even highly unusual behaviour would certainly not be regarded as mental illness, but, in any culture, some of the key features of the cases already cited would not be uncommon. Possession-like states can also arise as a result of intense mystical concentration and contemplation, coupled with deprivation of food, sleep, and deep or over-breathing. The life-styles and practices of some of the mystics of ancient days would tend to support such a contention. In some cultures, in parts of India, for example, where Tantric rites are practised (but disapproved of), sexual activities are used to heighten ecstatic awareness to produce trance-like conditions. It is of interest to note in this respect that sexually deviant conduct has often been associated with occult phenomena; in the twentieth century, the practices of occultists such as Aleister Crowley involved a wide range of sexually deviant conduct to assist them in their avowed search for 'truth'.

A number of possession-like states are to be found associated with some of the so-called 'culture-bound' syndromes that span the globe (see also Chapter four). In Japan, within the Ainu community, the shamans (priest-like figures) become possessed and give prophetic utterance. Anthropologists have suggested that a number of these shamans have psychological difficulties which they attempt to resolve through the possession trance.[19] In Nicaragua and in Honduras, amongst some of the village communities, there exists a condition described as *Grisi Siknis*, which sometimes reaches epidemic proportions. In this condition, young females are said to perform remarkable feats whilst in a trance-like state. These can include catching poisonous snakes with their bare hands. It is also said that various 'devils' seek out the more attractive of them and procure them for sexual purposes. They also may act violently towards others whilst in their trance-like condition. Treatment includes the use of herbal potions and careful attention to the prevention of noxious influences (pollutions) whilst the cure is taking place.[20] Amongst the Northern Algonkian Indians the phenomenon of Windigo psychosis is said to be well established. In this condition, an individual comes to believe he or she is possessed by a cannibalistic devil; in the course of such possession they may perform cannibalistic activities – for example, killing and eating the flesh of their victims. However, it needs to be pointed out that anthropologists appear to disagree as to the actual extent of this particular phenomenon.[21] In Singapore, a study was carried out of thirty-six young national servicemen referred to psychiatrists because of possession-type symptoms. They came from three different ethnic communities. At follow-up, some four to five years later, none of the twenty-six who could be traced showed any evidence of mental illness. Their strange behaviour was seen as a reaction to the stresses of engaging in service life. However, none was discharged from national service on medical grounds. This illustration is of interest for two reasons. First, because it suggests that there may well have been an element of mass suggestibility amongst these young men; second, because it demonstrates yet again, and in more modern guise, the mechanism through which supernatural forces may be used to claim exculpation from responsibility for things one finds not to one's liking or that are productive of stress.[22]

In parts of Egypt and in Ethiopia the phenomenon of Zar possession is not uncommon; in this phenomenon, trance-like states are fairly readily induced. In Haiti, Voodoo and its practices occur within a society in which poverty and a general air of depression may readily facilitate these practices in a vulnerable community. Voodoo and allied states have been summed up by Lewis as follows:

> Abreaction is the order of the day. Repressed urges and desires, the idiosyncratic as well as the socially conditioned are given public rein. No holds are barred. No interests are too unseemly in this setting not to receive sympathetic attention. Each dancer ideally achieves a state of ecstasy ... and collapses in a trance from which he emerges purged and refreshed.[23]

Finally, in completing this all too brief survey, an observation from a recent study of practices in India serves two useful purposes. First, it demonstrates the need for a multi-disciplinary approach to the problem of possession, and second, it serves as a useful lead-in to the next section of this chapter – the issue of differential diagnosis – that is of 'madness' or 'badness'.

> Patients consult psychiatrists after they have consulted a *pujari* (priest) and paid for a *puja* (worship service). In addition, they go back to the priests to have them perform mantras (chants) on the anti-psychotic medication they receive from the psychiatrists.... If the [treatment fails], then the priests may confine the patient to one of the special temples for various periods of time (up to 48 days) to expel the allegedly evil spirits or to undo the black magic.[24]

Differential diagnosis – madness or badness

From what has been described so far, it requires no great effort to discern that the boundaries between those states that would clearly be described as demonic and those ascribable to other causes are by no means clear cut. In Figure 3.1 I have tried to illustrate three possible groups of causative factors, but the cautionary note appended to the diagram should be constantly borne in mind. As we shall see, it is very important to try to make as good a differential diagnosis as possible so that management, by whatever means, may be effective. The point I am trying to make is illustrated by the following cases. One concerns the well-known case of a 31-year-old man who had allegedly become possessed. Following an all night exorcism he killed his wife in a particularly savage manner believing that she was troubled by an evil spirit. He was brought to trial, found to be suffering from a clear-cut, but fortunately short-lived, mental illness. Given appropriate medical treatment he was restored fairly quickly to his former state of good mental health. It was considered that the attempt at exorcism had served to precipitate his mental breakdown. Another concerned two priests in West Germany. They were charged with causing the death of a prostitute by starvation; believing her to be possessed they believed that such treatment was necessary to drive the devil out of her. In France, a woman described as a local sorceress had a farm labourer strapped to a bed and given nothing to eat but salt and water blessed by her in order to drive out the demons from him.[25] In another case, a mother and her two young children were killed by a man who believed he was possessed by the spirits of Chinese gods. He had almost completely severed the head of the children's mother, slit the throat of one child, and throttled the other. At his trial, he successfully pleaded not guilty to murder on the grounds of diminished responsibility and was ordered to be detained in a secure (Special) hospital without limit of time. At his trial, doctors testified that he suffered from a severe personality disorder and had six personalities believing he was possessed by different Chinese gods.[26] (See also the comments on multiple personality disorder in Chapter two.) The final illustration, rather like the case of the Yakima adolescent referred to earlier, shows that psychiatry may have little to offer in some instances. This was the case of a 38-year-old married woman who believed that while in a state of possession she had intercourse with the devil. Her local minister supported her in her beliefs and it appeared that treatment through prayer had helped her. She had refused medical treatment and, in the view of the psychiatrist who had been trying to help her, the diagnosis of her condition remained in some doubt.[27] These cases all illustrate the problem of the border-

Figure 3.1

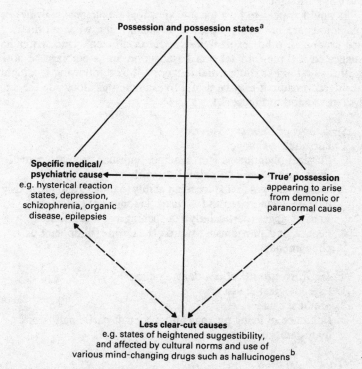

Possession and possession states[a]

Specific medical/
psychiatric cause
e.g. hysterical reaction
states, depression,
schizophrenia, organic
disease, epilepsies

'True' possession
appearing to arise
from demonic or
paranormal cause

Less clear-cut causes
e.g. states of heightened suggestibility,
and affected by cultural norms and use of
various mind-changing drugs such as hallucinogens[b]

Notes:
a   The dangers of trying to provide neat self-contained categories are obvious; the figure is thus
an over-simplification. The broken line indicates the interrelatedness of the possible causes
of the phenomena and also serves to emphasise the vital part played by socio-cultural factors.
b   Such drugs have included alcohol, mescaline, datura, and rauwolfia among others. The use of
mind-altering drugs is discussed again in Chapter five.

land already touched upon in this book. Such a borderland – between
sanity and insanity – is, of course, recognised in some societies; for
example, in the concept of 'Bardo' in the cult of Tibetan Tantrism.[28]
Reference has already been made to the casting out by Jesus of the
devil in the boy in the book of *Mark*. It is *possible*, of course, that epilepsy *may* have been the cause of the malady, but it has also been
suggested that epilepsy might have been but a symptom of a malady
of demonic origin.[29] The problematic borderline is further exemplified in the case of a man, diagnosed as suffering from schizophrenia,
who was troubled by demonic voices. In his case it was concluded that
he suffered from schizophrenia and demonic influence. An exorcism
was carried out and, subsequently, though still showing some schizo-

phrenic symptomatology, he was no longer troubled by his voices and intrusive thoughts.[30]

It would appear to be a tenable view that theological (Divine) explanations are necessary, because, in some cases, when all the facts are examined, other explanations seem insufficient. One writer has suggested a three-fold schema based upon an assemblage of authorities as an aid to differential diagnosis.[31] The following is a highly abridged version; it may be useful to examine this alongside the analysis presented in Figure 3.1.

Symptoms of Demonic 'Attack'
1. Personality change.
2. Physical phenomena (for example, unusual strength, convulsions, anaesthesia to painful stimuli).
3. Mental changes (evidence of an ability to understand previously unlearned languages and to speak 'in tongues' (glossolalia); voice changes (particularly a deepening and uncouthness).
4. Fear of, and antagonism towards, the Divine (blasphemous phenomena).

'False' Possession (but not denying its reality)
1. Psychological cause.
2. Medical cause.
3. Influence of living persons and by occult participation and manipulation.

'True' Possession
1. Due to occult experiences.
2. By invitation (active espousal of the Devil).
3. By unknown influence – mediumistic.

The important point to observe about any such schema is the degree of overlap and the arbitrary nature of any apparent neat categories.

Some further pointers

At this point it may be helpful to summarise some of the manifestations likely to be demonstrated by persons suffering from a variety of possession states – however categorised. These may include fits, fainting, contortion of the limbs, unusual strength, voice changes, violent dancing, a claim to clairvoyant powers, insensitivity to pain, vomiting, nausea, paralysis in varying degree, utterance of obscenities and blasphemies, an understanding of unlearned languages and a capacity to speak them, fear of the Divine presence, and rituals and regalia associated with it. One may well ask, how it is possible, with such an assemblage of disparate phenomena, to distinguish 'true' possession from other forms? The answer to this question is 'with considerable difficulty'. The truly possessed person, as distinct from the mentally ill individual, despite being very restless, may remain 'sane' in most other areas of his or her thinking. Mentally ill persons may tend to talk a good deal about their 'demons'; the truly possessed tend to avoid discussion of such matters unless directly approached upon the topic. The voices heard by the truly possessed will not have the incongruity often found in the mentally ill. In addition, care needs to be taken in distinguishing the degree to which a person appearing to be experiencing possession is suffering from the passivity feelings experienced by some schizophrenics. In such cases, the person feels that others may be taking them over. True possession states are also likely to be more transient than schizophrenic illnesses. The truly possessed will be less likely to be conscious of their state of mind and will not be disturbed by blasphemous thoughts and utterances in the way that a mentally ill person may be disturbed and distressed by them.[32] Some clues may be afforded in answer to questions put to a patient such as 'Why are you, or do you feel yourself to be, possessed?' As has already been indicated, conventional psychiatric and other disorders may exist alongside demonic phenomena. Sims puts the matter very succinctly: 'a Satanist who contracts pneumonia following the celebration of a wintry Sabbath requires antibiotics; the symptoms of psychotic depression will demand apropriate treatment with anti-depressant drugs or electro-convulsive therapy.'[33] This last point is important because, in depressive disorders, feelings of being controlled or influenced by evil or Satanic forces are not uncommon; and it would be unfortunate to overlook a true depressive illness and the chance of treating it with the effective means now at our disposal. This is why it is vital for all who work in this area – whether they be a doctor, priest or informed lay worker – to take a careful and full social and personal history.[34] Such a history will also help the worker to clarify the degree to which involvement in such practices as experimentation with ouija boards, Tarot-like interpretations, other forms of clairvoyance and contact with other apparatus of the occult, may have heightened the susceptibility of an already vulnerable person. The remarks made earlier about the contemporary interest in, and dabbling with, the occult are highly relevant here.

To conclude this section, a statement of what seventeenth-century and earlier writers had to say about differential diagnosis may be of interest since a number of the signs are also to be found in more modern writings. It was suggested that there were eleven indicators of true possession:

1. To think oneself possessed
2. To lead a wicked life
3. To live outside the rules of society
4. To be persistently ill, falling into heavy sleep, and vomiting unusual objects (either natural objects: toads, serpents, worms, iron, stones, etc; or artificial objects: nails, pins, etc which may also be illusions caused by witches and not inevitably signs of possession by the devil)
5. To blaspheme
6. To make a pact with the devil
7. To be troubled with spirits ('an absolute and inner possession and residence in the body of the person')
8. To show a frightening and horrible countenance
9. To be tired of living (*s'ennuyer de vivre et se désespérer*)
10. To be uncontrollable and violent
11. To make sounds and movements like an animal

These indications should alert the priest for the *sure signs* of demoniacal possession: revealing secret and hidden information; speaking or comprehending strange languages; displaying phenomenal strength and extraordinary body movements; and reacting to sacred objects (italics in original).[35]

Deliverance (exorcism/healing)

It needs to be re-emphasised that it is highly advisable for anyone dealing with a possession state to keep an open mind as to its causality. This presupposes a flexibility of approach and a capacity for the disciplines of medicine and theology to come together for a common purpose – namely the relief of suffering. It is obviously important to rule out as far as possible the presence of treatable mental illness as a first step (but, as already suggested, it is equally important to recognise the possibility of the presence of co-existing phenomena). Equally important is the need to involve friends and relations in the process of healing and after-care. The latter is especially important in cases where attempts are being made to wean someone away from occult and allied influences. Of equal importance is the need for those who counsel in this area to have both emotional and physical support in this very draining task – as already noted, the risk of feeling contaminated is very high. It is not a task to be undertaken lightly by any counsellor, particularly the lay man or woman. It may not surprise readers to know that writing this chapter has not only been a difficult intellectual task, but the nature of the material I have had to research into (and only reported upon briefly here) has had a considerable emotional impact upon me. If a formal rite of exorcism is decided upon, the simpler it is kept the better. The form of words to be used varies depending upon the particular church affiliation of the person officiating. All of them seem to embody in one form or another the simple adjuration to the force possessing the person (1) to do no harm; (2) to emerge; (3) to depart. One form of words suggested in a Church of England report on exorcism suggests the following: 'that harming no-one, you depart from this creature of God ... and return to the place appointed you, there to remain for ever'.[36] As with all forms of therapeutic endeavour, much depends upon the faith and confidence of the person carrying out the rite – whether it be merely the use of words or by the additional laying on of hands, or whether it be accompanied by the use of holy water or other physical rituals.[37]

Conclusions

Whether dealing with states of so-called possession or true neurosis, the need to recognise the power of suggestion, on the part of both the healer or priest and the afflicted, is paramount. As we have seen, this and the culture and social environment in which the afflicted person lives, the use of drugs or other stimulants, may induce some forms of possession. Some may be possessed by God or by Satan, by the spirits of ancestors, or by Allah, or by a wide range of supernatural agents. William Sargent, after researching the phenomena in many parts of the world, was forced to conclude as follows:

I think I might have to end these long years of research with the conclusion that there are no gods, but only impressions of gods created in man's mind, so varied are the gods and creeds which have been brought into being by playing on emotional arousal, increased suggestibility and abnormal phases of brain activity.[38]

Sargent seems to be leaving out the possibility of some Divine force and this would be in keeping with his cautious and somewhat sceptical approach to these matters. In my view, every age appears to have its need to find its own 'devils'. Freudian and other psychoanalytic schools of thought would see them as a means of dealing with our repressed desires and wishes and of hating the unholy and unhealthy parts of ourselves in others. A Jungian perspective lends considerable credence to the notion that we all have a hidden or darker side. It is not surprising, therefore, that we seem to need to find a variety of accessible repositories for our hates and fears. Anyone who shows a departure from the norm is likely to inspire such distorted fear-ridden beliefs. Witches and their like have, to some extent, been replaced by other 'alien' beings; outsiders, such as Jews, people of dark skin, gypsies, the mentally ill, and the handicapped. To which, of course, must be added the criminal and, more recently, those suffering from auto-immune deficiency disease. As I write these words, we are currently projecting our fears on to less animate scapegoats such as eggs and cheese! There appears to be no end to the extent to which men and women have to find vehicles for the projection of their anxieties and guilt.

Notes and references

1. P.M. Yap, 'The Possession Syndrome: A Comparison of Hong Kong and French Findings', *Journal of Mental Science*, 1960, vol. 106, pp. 114–137.
2. J. Richards, *But Deliver Us From Evil: An Introduction to the Demonic Dimension in Pastoral Care*, London, Darton, Longman and Todd, 1984.
3. Richards, op. cit. 1984, p. 91.
4. See B. Walker, *Encyclopaedia of Metaphysical Medicine*, London, Routledge and Kegan Paul, 1978, p. 221.
5. A useful summary of this work may be found in M. Summers, *The Geography of Witchcraft*, London, Routledge and Kegan Paul, 1927 (Reprinted 1978), pp. 477–479.
6. I.M. Lewis, *Ecstatic Religion: An Anthropological Study of Spirit Possession and Shamanism*, Harmondsworth, Penguin Books, 1971, p. 31.
7. See, for example, S. Kemp, 'Modern Myth and Mediaeval Madness: Views of Mental Illness in the European Middle Ages and Renaissance', *New Zealand Journal of Psychology*, 1985, vol. 14, pp. 1–8. Also, S. Kemp and H. Williams, 'Demonic Possession and Mental Disorder in Early Modern Europe', *Psychological Medicine*, 1987, vol. 17, pp. 21–29. A description of a case of ecstatic possession in a thirteenth-century adolescent may be found in J. Kroll and R. de Ganck, 'The Adolescence of a Thirteenth-century Visionary Nun', *Psychological Medicine*, 1986, vol. 16, pp. 745–756. For discussions of the age-old problem of the relationship between the development of scientific thought and religious beliefs see W. James, *Varieties of Religious Experience: A Study of Human Nature*, London, Longman, 1902. Further useful titles may be found in R. Porter, *A Social History of Madness: Stories of the Insane*, London, Weidenfeld and Nicolson, 1987, pp. 241–242. The most comprehensive discussion of the wider background is that by K. Thomas, *Religion and the Decline of Magic: Studies in Popular Beliefs in Sixteenth- and Seventeenth-century England*, Harmondsworth, Penguin Books, 1973 (especially at pp. 570–576). The relationship between the burgeoning of scientific thought, the mystical, and the occult is discussed very thoroughly in B. Vickers (ed.), *Occult and Scientific Mentalities in the*

Renaissance, Cambridge, Cambridge University Press (especially the Introduction and Chapters 3 and 12). A broad sociological context for the study of theories of magic is to be found in D.L. O'Keefe, *Stolen Lightning*, Oxford, Martin Robertson, 1982 (notably at pp. 414–457). For more general discussions of witchcraft see: M. Marwick (ed.), *Witchcraft and Sorcery: Selected Readings*, Harmondsworth, Penguin Books, 1982; H.R. Trevor-Roper, *The European Witch-craze of the Sixteenth and Seventeenth Centuries*, Harmondsworth, Penguin Books, 1978. The numerous mass epidemics of so-called possession that occurred between 1491 and 1749 are enumerated in R.H. Robbins, *The Encyclopaedia of Witchcraft and Demonology*, London, Newnes Books, 1984, pp. 393–394.

8. G.A. German, 'Mental Health in Africa (II): The Nature of Mental Disorder in Africa Today: Some Clinical Observations', *British Journal of Psychiatry*, 1987, vol. 151, pp. 440–446.

   A selection of approaches to possession states from anthropological, medical, theological, and sociological perspectives may be found in the following works:

   (a) E. Bourguignon, *Possession*, San Francisco, Chandler and Sharp, 1976

   (b) V. Crapanzano and V. Garrison, *Case Studies in Spirit Possession*, New York, Wiley, 1977

   (c) R.H. Cox (ed.), *Religious Systems and Psychotherapy*, Springfield, Illinois, C.C. Thomas, 1973

   (d) W.W. Eaton, *The Sociology of Mental Disorders* (2nd edn), New York, Praeger, 1986, Chapter 1

   (e) M.D. Enoch and W.H. Trethowan, *Uncommon Psychiatric Syndromes* (2nd edn), Bristol, Wright and Sons, 1979, Chapter 10

   (f) S. Freud, 'A Seventeenth-century Demonological Neurosis', in *Collected Works*, London, Hogarth Press, 1961

   (g) T.K. Osterreich, *Possession: Demoniacal and Other Among Primitive Races in Antiquity, the Middle Ages and Modern Times*, New York, New York University Press, 1966

   (h) M. Perry (ed.), *Deliverance: Psychic Disturbances and Occult Involvement*, London, SPCK, 1987

9. R. Storm, 'The Black Magic Games that Turn into Terror', *Independent*, 18 October 1988. In a more recent illustration of what appears to be a disturbing trend, a schoolboy was given an indeterminate sentence for a hammer attack upon a 28-year-old female teacher. He is said to have told the authorities that he was 'possessed by the Holy Spirit, could speak in tongues and was guided by God'. A psychiatrist told the court that the youth was severely psychiatrically disturbed and needed prolonged treatment (*Leicester Mercury*, 11 July 1989).

10. *The Times*, 25 August 1986.

11. All the quotations are taken from *The New English Bible With the*

Apocrypha (2nd edn), Oxford and Cambridge University Presses, 1970. For an interpretation of the meanings to be attached to biblical accounts see, for example, S.J. Wright, *Our Mysterious God*, Basingstoke, Marshalls, 1984, notably Chapter 2.

12. Quoted in W. Sargent, *The Mind Possessed: A Physiology of Possession, Mysticism and Faith Healing*, Ashford, Kent, Headley Brothers, 1985, p. 63.
13. Sargent, op. cit. 1985, p. 64.
14. Ibid., p. 65.
15. Ibid., p. 64.
16. Ibid., p. 66.
17. Sargent, op. cit.
18. E.M. Pattison, 'Possession States and Exorcism', in C.T.M. Friedmann and R.A. Faguet (eds), *Extraordinary Disorders of Human Behaviour*, New York, Plenum Books, 1982.
19. See E. Ohnuki-Tierney, 'Shamans and Imu Among Two Ainu Groups – Towards a Cross-cultural Model of Interpretation', in R.C. Simons and C.C. Hughes (eds), *The Culture-bound Syndromes: Folk Illnesses of Psychiatric and Anthropological Interest*, Lancaster, D. Reidel, 1985, pp. 91–110.
20. See P.A. Dennis, 'Grisi Siknis in Miskito Culture', in Simons and Hughes, op. cit. 1985, pp. 289–306.
21. See L. Marano, 'Windigo Psychosis: The Anatomy of an Emic-Etic Confusion', in Simons and Hughes, op. cit. 1985, pp. 411–448. A useful and cautious anthropological psychiatric approach to these and allied matters may be found in R. Littlewood, 'Russian Dolls and Chinese Boxes: An Anthropological Approach to the Implicit Models of Comparative Psychiatry', in J.L. Cox (ed.), *Transcultural Psychiatry*, London, Croom Helm, 1986, pp. 37–58. See also A. Kiev, *Transcultural Psychiatry*, Harmondsworth, Penguin, 1972, and more recently, P. Rack, *Race, Culture and Mental Disorder*, London, Tavistock, 1982.
22. E.H. Lua, L.P. Sin and K.T. Chee, 'A Cross-cultural Study of the Possession Trance in Singapore', *Australian and New Zealand Journal of Psychiatry*, 1986, vol. 20, pp. 361–364.
23. Lewis, op. cit. 1971, p. 195.
24. S.G. Mestrovic, 'Magic and Psychiatric Commitment in India', *International Journal of Law and Psychiatry*, 1986, vol. 9, pp. 431–449. The need for co-operation between psychiatrists and faith-healers is stressed in a paper by M.S. Keshavan, H.S. Narayanan and B.N. Gangadhar, '"Bhanamati" Sorcery and Psychopathology in South India: A Clinical Study', *British Journal of Psychiatry*, 1989, vol. 154, pp. 218–220. One writer has recently gone so far as to suggest that mystical and allied states are not within the realm of psychiatry. See A.J. Pelosi, 'The Mystical-ecstatic and Trance States', Letter, *British Journal of Psychiatry*, 1988, vol. 153, p. 412.
25. Cases described in Enoch and Trethowan, op. cit. 1979, Chapter 10.
26. *Independent*, 14 November 1987.

27. P.H. Salmons and D.J. Clarke, 'Cacedomonomania', *Psychiatry*, 1987, vol. 50, pp. 50–54.
28. See A.R. Favazza, *Bodies Under Siege: Self-mutilation in Culture and Society*, London, Johns Hopkins University Press, 1987, pp. 10–11.
29. Richards, op. cit. 1984, p. 103.
30. Richards, op. cit. 1984, p. 111.
31. Richards, op. cit. 1984, pp. 156–158.
32. Richards, ibid.
33. A. Sims, 'Demon Possession: Medical Perspective in a Western Culture', in B. Palmer (ed.), *Medicine and the Bible*, Exeter, The Paternoster Press (for the Christian Medical Fellowship), 1986, pp. 179–180. The chapter by Professor Sims makes a significant contribution to the role of psychiatry in dealing with possession disorders.
34. The need for this and other very useful practical points may be found in J. Allan, *Dealing With Darkness: The Church's Pastoral Response to the Occult*, Edinburgh, Handsell Press, 1986.
35. Robbins, op. cit. 1984, p. 395.
36. Richards, op. cit. 1984, p. 167. See also Dom R. Petitpierre, OSB (ed.), *Exorcism: The Findings of a Commission Convened by the Bishop of Exeter*, London, SPCK, 1972.
37. Details of the various forms of prayer and practice used in the rite of exorcism, including that of the Roman Catholic Church (Rituale Romanum) may be found in Robbins, op. cit. 1984, pp. 180–189.
38. Sargent, op. cit. 1985, p. 239.

Chapter four

Some so-called culture-bound syndromes

'I'll put a girdle round about the earth ...'
(*A Midsummer Night's Dream*, Act II, Scene i)

Introduction

In this chapter consideration is given to some illustrations of the so-called *culture-bound syndromes*. These consist of highly unusual forms of behaviour that, upon first inspection, often appear to be indigenous to particular cultures. However, as we shall see, there appears to be considerable disagreement among anthropologists and psychiatrists as to whether or not this is really the case. Many of the so-called culture-bound disorders appear to be found in ethnically diverse cultures including European communities. The dispute concerning their indigenous existence merely illustrates once again the need for a multi-disciplinary and inter-national approach to the subject. Some anthropologists have suggested two useful conceptual approaches to the topic. The first consists of *-emic* explanations; these cover indigenous cultural accounts (such as the actions of witches or other 'evil' folk). The second deals with *-etic* explanations; these include the use of the episode or phenomenon as a legitimate sick role for the victim. This serves as a means of institutionalised tension resolution and as a temporary release from stressful situations (see, for example, the psychiatric explanations given for some 'possession' states described in Chapter three).[1] Such approaches help to demonstrate how anthropology seeks to make links between psychopathology and culture. It is worthy of comment that, apart from one or two notable exceptions, there are very few psychiatrists formally trained in the discipline of anthropology.[2] Some authorities indicate that certain phenomena, such as amok, can only be understood within a specific cultural framework;[3] others consider that amok is peculiar to Malaya. Thus: 'The stereotypic amok pattern is clearly labelled in Malaya, pertains to concepts of masculine honour specific to the area and as such pre-exists any specific manifestations of it.'[4] An alternative view is that culture-bound syndromes may be seen as examples of mental disorders that do not fit easily into our western systems of classification; for this reason they have been 'thought to be specific to a particular culture'.[5] A contrary perspective has been expressed in the following terms: 'culture-bound disorders are for the most part variants of the severe functional psychoses and of the various neurotic syndromes ... they are not new diagnostic entities; they are in fact similar to those already known in the West.'[6] In concluding this brief introduction it is important to remember that we should be as precise as possible in our use of terminology, even though the evidence strongly in favour of one approach or another is somewhat inconclusive. In this connection, the influence of the media upon public attitudes is of considerable importance, particularly in western societies which are now becoming increasingly ethnically diverse. A study of public attitudes in the wake of Michael Ryan's mass killings at Hungerford makes this point very clearly. In this retrospective survey of public attitudes towards the relationship between mental illness and violence the authors of this study found a significant increase in the number of persons believing that those who commit senseless and horrific crimes are likely to be mentally ill. However, they found no change in the proportion of those believing that the mentally ill are likely to be more violent. The authors concluded that as the true mental state of Ryan was unknown (see pp. 48–50) speculation by the press and psychiatrists may have resulted in this change without influencing the public view of mental illness in general.[7] We can now consider a selection of so-called culture-bound syndromes, and particular those of *amok* and *koro*.

Amok

Background

In our culture, amok-like states are sometimes characterised by loss of contact with reality, accompanying excitement, and gross disinhibition. We use the term amok to describe sudden eruptions of 'random destructiveness, usually of psychogenic origin'.[8]

The evidence suggests that in all cultures there appears to be a strongly dissociative element, which seems to produce a capacity for mass killing and a subsequent amnesia for the events amongst those who survive. (Similar dissociative phenomena are, of course, sometimes seen in those who have carried out serial killings over a long period of time.) The word 'amok' (also known as *amock* or *amuck*) is a Malay expression denoting homicidal assault. It has a long and world-wide history and appears to have been described most frequently in Malaya and India and more frequently reported upon by psychiatrists and anthropologists. However, it is also seen in many other parts of the world; for example, Singapore, Australia, Canada, Japan, Siberia, Kenya, New Guinea, and the United States. Various other names have been used to describe the phenomenon in some of these countries; in the Sahara, as *pseudonite*, in Polynesia as *cathard*, in Canada as the 'Jumping Frenchman' phenomenon and in the U.S.A. as the 'Whitman syndrome'. One of the earliest descriptions of the condition is that given by Nicolo Conti in the 1430s.[9] Westermeyer[10] has suggested that the word has now taken on a more general usage and that lay men and women have tended to use it to apply to any sudden and dramatic outbreaks of random violence. In Scandinavia, in ancient times, such behaviour was seen amongst warriors in battle and known as 'berserk', hence the common and somewhat erroneous use of the word in more modern times. In its clinical presentation it seems to begin with a period of social isolation and withdrawal from others. The person described as *amok* would then suddenly attack anyone within easy reach such as friends, family, or innocent strangers; multiple killings would be frequent. Such assaults would continue until the amok was finally killed, killed himself, or was restrained by force. Those who survived would fall into a profound sleep or semi-coma of varying duration. Following return to wakefulness there would almost invariably be amnesia for the event. According to some observers there would also be a period of depression in some cases. The manifestation appears to have been observed in most social classes and occupations. It is significant, however, that its perpetrators are usually, but not exclusively, male, single, divorced, or separated.

It has been suggested that the phenomenon known as *latah* (which includes amongst other things the shouting of vulgarities and obscenities) can be regarded in some respects as the female equivalent of amok. Some authorities use the term *mengamok* to mean the act of running amok and *pengamok* to indicate the person who actually runs amok. Cultural historians have noted that cries of 'amok, amok' were common in the heat of battle in ancient times and were used as a means of instilling fear into one's foes. Throughout all the studies that have been made the phenomenon of isolation appears to be very common as is the presence of some self-defined 'insult'.[11] Weapons used in amok attacks have included short swords (keris), guns (in more developed societies), batons, hatchets – almost any instrument that easily comes to hand and is capable of inflicting serious injury. One writer has suggested that 'its sudden ... onset is usually due to the fact that previous symptoms of distress have gone un-noticed rather than to their sudden appearance'.[12] (See also p. 51.)

Some attempts at explanation

Partly because of the somewhat random manner in which samples of such behaviour have been collected over the years, numerous and sometimes conflicting observations on causation have been reported. Early investigators suggested 'biomedical causal factors'.[13] Among these were neurosyphilis, malaria, typhoid, leprosy, epilepsy, and poisoning. In more recent years psychodynamic factors have been considered as important; during the past decade or two a multi-causal approach has found most favour in which the phenomenon has been described in individual psychopathological terms but located clearly within socio-cultural networks. The need to study the social context is certainly vitally important. Although the phenomenon is seen by some as a form of brief reactive psychosis the true picture is likely to be much more complex than this. Amok has been described by an anthropologically trained psychiatrist as a 'final common pathway along which are channelled various kinds of problem: acute and chronic psychoses ... but also criminal behaviour without psychopathology, alcohol and drug induced states and so forth'.[14] This author also stresses the importance of the social context and advises caution in trying to determine whether a phenomenon is evidence of mental disturbance or not. He uses response to bereavement as an example:

> the determination of whether such reports are a sign of an abnormal mental state is an interpretation based on knowledge of the ... group's behavioural norms ... hearing the voice of the dead is an expected experience ... in bereavement ... among a number of American Indian tribal groups; this experience does not portend psychosis ... to interpret these normal experiences as 'hallucinations' with all the significance of pathology the term connotes is ... *not valid*. (Italics in original.)[15]

In this context, one is mindful of the need not to 'pathologise' behaviour that may be 'normal' in our increasingly ethnically diverse society.

For example, some Afro-Caribbeans may customarily speak to God and hear God speaking directly to them. For them, this may be a quite 'normal' experience and is not necessarily to be taken as a manifestation of psychosis by the unwary and uninformed western psychiatric professional. In the paper just quoted, Kleinman goes on to suggest that one of the most useful roles for anthropology in relation to psychiatry is to challenge attempts 'to medicalise the human condition, to encourage humility in the face of alternative cultural formulation of human problems ... and to make us uncomfortable with our taken-for-granted professional categories'.[16] In such a context, therefore, the phenomenon of amok may not necessarily be regarded as 'a disease, but rather a behavioural sequence that may be precipitated by a number of aetiological factors, among them physical, psychological as well as socio-cultural determinants'.[17] Accounts from folk-lore point to possession by evil spirits, breaking of taboos, and other magical influences as causal agents. Psychodynamic interpretations have stressed the need to project blame (by way of imagined wrongs and self-defined insults) on to others. The need to control anger (until a crisis makes it erupt) is a paramount theoretical consideration, as is over-sensitivity to imagined hurts. Such paranoid-type feelings may be very important factors. It would also appear that many people who indulge in amok-type behaviour have problems in establishing relationships and they also find difficulty in expressing hostility. As already noted, they are 'loners' and have poor pre-morbid personalities. Certainly loss of self-esteem, being placed in deeply embarrassing situations by others, or in a state of apparently unresolvable crisis seem significant factors in the backgrounds of those who exhibit such behaviour. In some studies, the phenomenon appears to be regarded as *endemic*; that is, it does not appear to be alien to prevailing culture which may, in fact, facilitate it. In others, it would appear to be *epidemic*; that is, it appears to be a reaction to temporary phases of crisis, is not so frequent, and has no apparent established tradition. Some authorities have suggested that the notion of an ethnic unconscious is useful by way of explanation. In some ways, this may appear similar to the concept of the collective unconscious formulated by Carl Jung. The ethnic unconscious

is that portion of the total unconscious segment of the individual psyche which is shared with most members of a given culture in that ... society or culture permits certain impulses, fantasies and the like to become and to remain conscious, while requiring others to be repressed. The members of a given culture are likely to have repressed the same things and thereby to have certain unconscious conflicts in common.[18]

Working towards a classification

Westermeyer has suggested that the amok syndrome can be defined as SMASH (Sudden Mass Assault Syndrome With Homicide).[19] The criteria for such a designation would include the following:

1. a sudden outburst of violent behaviour (the violence may have been thought about or planned for some time, but the actual violent behaviour should be sudden and unexpected);
2. a public display of the violence, so that the perpetrator allows himself/herself to be readily identified in the community;
3. the injurious behaviour should not be specifically aimed at only one or a few people, but should occur against all present;
4. the community should not support the violence, so that the perpetrator is restrained, executed, exiled or imprisoned ... ;
5. at least one or more homicides ensue from the assault (this arbitrary criterion will limit the cases to those most dangerous and serious).

The criterion that includes slaughter in large numbers is important. The thinking that may lie behind such mayhem has been graphically described as follows:

> In other words, if you are driven to slaughter, slay as many people as you can; the more you kill, the more you will be remembered. This is the spirit of the 'amok' ... the man who elects 'amok' is beyond the canons of human reason.[20]

Burton-Bradley has made extensive studies of amok-like behaviour, particularly in the communities of Papua New Guinea.[21] He has recently reported upon seven cases showing some of the characteristics referred to earlier; in so doing he describes feelings that may frequently lie behind this often incomprehensible form of behaviour, and he also notes in passing that his presentation is a form of cultural paraphrase:

> I am not an important 'big man'. I possess only my personal dignity. My life has been reduced to nothing by an intolerable insult. Therefore, I have nothing to lose except my life, which is nothing, so I trade my life for yours, as your life is favoured. The exchange is in my favour, so I shall not only kill you, but I shall kill many of you, and at the same time rehabilitate myself in the eyes of the group of which I am a member, even though I might be killed in the process.[22]

Burton-Bradley suggests that behind such thinking lies a state of hypereredism (a state of hostile morbid tension).[23] This can lead to the explosive behaviour already described, which is *out of all propor-*

tion to the circumstances. He suggests a hard-core symptomatology in all such cases, based upon the self-defined insult. Four discrete periods may be discerned: '(a) a prodromal brooding, during which a resolution may be effected if circumstances permit; (b) explosive homicidal outburst; (c) continuing homicidal drive; and (d) a retrospective claim of amnesia by the ones who survive.' He cites two recent cases by way of illustration; in so doing he suggests that the increased activity to ban firearms will not *of itself* reduce the incidence of such events; he suggests that emotive coverage by the media may merely serve to make matters worse.[24] (See also the discussion of media treatment, p. 43.) Some of the aetiological and presenting characteristics already identified have been supported in recent work by the forensic psychiatrist, Arboleda-Florez.[25] In a description of four mass assault cases he too emphasises the loneliness, social isolation, withdrawal, and brooding behind the perpetration of these apparently motiveless homicides. One of the cases was that of the Calgary Mall sniper who was charged with the attempted murder of 8 people. The others are those of Charles Whitman, who killed 13 and wounded 31, Unruh, the 49-year-old who, in 1949, killed 13, and a Canadian man of 22 who, in 1972, killed 3 and wounded 7 others. This author emphasises the importance of the feelings of alienation and a need for assertiveness (based, one imagines, on past faulty development) and a social factor, namely that of living in a society in a time of transition and change. The latter experience is likely to be particularly stressful for those who feel a need to cultivate a 'macho' image based upon Rambo-like cult figures and who feel pushed aside in a society that is increasingly governed by competitiveness and who feel a need to demonstrate overt success. It is obviously important to differentiate amok-like assaults from serial murder and from acts of terrorism. Both of these are usually well planned and well carried out activities; the motivation is likely to be more clearly discernible. In terms of current psychiatric classification the phenomenon of amok perhaps may be regarded as similar to a brief reactive psychosis or isolated explosive disorder;[26] it would seem to fit the SMASH syndrome already described.

Michael Ryan and some other cases

The case of Michael Ryan was referred to briefly in the opening pages of this book. We can now consider this case in a little more detail. Ryan was aged 27 at the time of the tragic events that occurred in the small market town of Hungerford.[27] He had been described as a 'wimp' at school and a 'loner'. His mother apparently doted upon him. Doubtless he may have felt a degree of ambivalence about such devotion but, faced with the lack of detail about their relationship, it would seem to have been unwise to have indulged in the theorising about the causal implications of the relationship that appeared in the press at the time of the tragedy (see Chapter one). He left school at 16 with no real accomplishments to his name and took 'dead-end' jobs. He is said to have been without success in his relationships with the opposite sex, but made up stories about his conquests and is said to have created a fictional fiancée. He also created several fictional friends who he suggested were people of considerable influence. Significantly, he had a short spell helping at a gun-shop and was a licensed member of a gun club. His period of mayhem seems to have started at about 12.40 a.m. on the day in question and to have continued till about 7 p.m. that night when, finally, he killed himself (having apparently expressed regret at having killed his mother). His mass killings appear to have been quite random and they included the slaughter of a mother of two small children – this was carried out in front of them.

He used a powerful AK 47 rifle – a particularly deadly weapon but, as has already been suggested, any other readily available weapon would, in the circumstances, have been equally lethal. One interesting speculation seems to have emerged at the inquest. In respect of the murder of the mother of the two children it was suggested that a sexual motive might have been possible since he forced her to take a ground-sheet from the boot of her car with them. One elderly witness described her impression of him at the inquest as follows:

> He had a terrible vacant look in his eyes and a funny sort of grin on his face. He looked as if he was brain dead. I had known him for over 20 years, but he was so strange that I didn't recognise him.[28]

The final picture we have of Ryan was that of a body with 'his pistol, tied to his wrist by a cord ... cocked and loaded with six rounds of ammunition; around the body were scattered the debris of his phantasy world, a 9 mm magazine, a pair of handcuffs and a kit for cleaning guns'.[29]

As Ryan did not live to be questioned about his life and motives and as little, if anything, has ever emerged about his history from any other source, we can only conjecture as to whether his behaviour was a form of classical amok. Certainly he seems to have exhibited some, but not all, of the key features. He exhibited loneliness, isolation and a low level of competence and, perhaps more speculatively, low self-esteem in a world that seems to set such a premium upon competence and observable success. His attack was sudden, we may imagine it to be fairly unpremeditated, but this is perhaps question-able. He suffered death at his own hand, a feature not universally characteristic of amok. I would not be averse to speculating a little further that he had been brooding on his poor performance and pres-entation for some considerable time. This may have driven him to his final explosive cataclysmic outburst – 'in for a penny, in for a pound, I'll be somebody at last'. One can only speculate as to whether it would have been possible for a professional 'listener' to have inter-vened with positive effect had one been given the chance. We know from other tragedies that such opportunities are sadly sometimes missed.

Four further cases

These four cases, reported upon briefly, are included in an attempt to fill out the picture, but it is not claimed that they adequately illustrate all aspects of classical amok-like behaviour.

The first is of a school-teacher aged 36. He admitted manslaughter (on the grounds of diminished responsibility) of two people and was found guilty of the attempted murder of two others. He had become obsessed with a teenage boy – the son of one of his victims and had threatened to do 'something like Hungerford' as a result of his obses-sion. Three months later he put his plans into effect when he was posted to another school and thus parted from the object of his obsession. (There is no evidence in the reports of this case that this was in any sense a physical relationship.) Although obviously not a description of classic amok, the case certainly demonstrates the powerful and all-pervasive effect of brooding in such cases.[30]

The second case is that of James Huberty, aged 41, married with two children. In July 1984, he walked into a Macdonalds in a small town in Southern California and shot dead 20 people and wounded 20 more. Significantly, he had for long been regarded as an 'outsider' in his own community.[31]

The third brief example concerns a 19-year-old from Melbourne. He killed 6 people and injured 18 before he allegedly ran out of am-munition. It is noteworthy that he too was something of an outsider; he was said to have been a 'drop-out' from a military academy.[32]

Sadly, as I write this chapter, a further serious incident has been reported from the quiet suburb of Monkseaton, near Whitley Bay in northern England. At about 12 noon on Sunday 30 April 1989, Robert Sartin, a 22-year-old civil servant, in a fourteen-minute out-burst, shot dead a 41-year-old man and caused injuries to 13 others; 11 victims were taken to hospital with shotgun wounds and 2 others were reported as being hurt by flying glass. First reports of the incident indicated that 3 of those who were in hospital were said to be in a serious condition. The assailant was subsequently charged with the murder of the 41-year-old man. Dressed apparently entirely in black, and wearing sun-glasses, the man walked through several streets firing indiscriminately from a 12-bore shotgun. He was eventually tackled by an unarmed policeman who gave chase in an unmarked police car. No apparent motive for the outburst is currently available and the victims were said to be unknown to the assailant. He was described by more than one observer as calm, cold, robot-like, offering no resistance when arrested. He is said to have made one interesting and maybe revealing remark to one of his potential victims – an elderly woman. He pointed his gun at her and said 'I won't shoot you – you're too old.'[33]

Summary

It is difficult to find conclusive evidence that amok-like behaviour is essentially culture-bound; i.e. that its manifestation is essentially dependent upon local circumstances and traditions. However, the earlier descriptions of the condition provided by anthropologists and psychiatrists do seem to indicate indigenous features in some cases. Common characteristics of the syndrome would seem to include the following: normally being young, male, single, divorced or separated and showing a degree of abnormal introspection and isolation. In addition, there exists a strong and highly pervasive feeling of resentment at injustices (self-defined insults). All these may result in explosive homicidal behaviour which is directed non-specifically at a variety of victims. More often than not the behaviour ends in the death of the assailant. This occurs either at the hands of the authorities in a legitimated killing or by suicide. Thus, in many cases, we are deprived of opportunities to examine in any detail not only whether our speculations as to motivation have any substance, but, perhaps of equal importance, what measures might be successful in treatment and/or prevention. This fact is, perhaps, of particular significance when one considers the 'copy-cat' cases that often seem to occur after a notorious case has 'hit the headlines'. Two such cases (in Bristol and Walsall) appear to have occurred after the Hungerford case. The fact that some people have been brooding quietly and ominously on their imagined, or even real, injustices for very long periods of time is an extremely worrying one. Such brooding has, for one reason or another, defied recognition; this must be very troubling to both professional care-givers and to the public alike. There is little doubt in my mind that, admittedly on hindsight, patterns do emerge and clues are sometimes missed.

In the next section of this chapter brief consideration is given to a rather different form of behaviour, which, if not immediately life-threatening to the general public, is certainly very distressing to the sufferer. It is also on first sight a very bizarre form of behaviour.

Koro (Shook Yang) – genital retraction syndrome

It is not uncommon for people suffering from a variety of mental disorders to claim that their bodily functions are severely impaired and/or to believe that their vital organs have been damaged in some way. Such phenomena may be found most noticeably in schizophrenic disorder,[34] but also in melancholia and in certain organic conditions. From time to time individuals may present with variants of the monosymptomatic disorders described in Chapter two. In such presentations the cardinal characteristics may be perceptual delusions about bodily function and appearance. One such disorder is that commonly described as *koro*. As we shall see, the koro or *genital retraction syndrome* illustrates, yet again, the problems inherent in trying to classify such disorders satisfactorily within a conventional psychiatric framework; they illustrate also the extent to which such disorders can or cannot be regarded entirely as culture specific. Currently there appears to be no uniform view about this matter and this is well documented in a recent review of the topic.[35]

The use of the term

There is considerable speculation as to the exact derivation of the word 'koro'. It has been traced to the Javanese word for 'tortoise' because of its similarity to the *glans penis*. Others have suggested that the word is derived from a Malay term *Keruk* – to shrink. The Chinese variant of the word is *Shook Y(o)ang* (Suk-Yeong) meaning literally shrinking penis.[36]

Major characteristics and presentation

Koro has been described as an 'acute hysterical panic reaction, brought on by auto- or hetero-suggestion and conditioned by the cultural background' of the sufferer.[37] The cultural context has been further emphasised in the following way: 'It would appear that the disease is probably a result of free play of imagination of a physician on top of a culture which links fatality with genital retraction and sexual activity with risk to life.'[38] The key characteristic of the disorder is the belief that the penis is retracting into the abdomen. In some parts of the world, notably in China, the disorder has also been characterised by a second and important belief, namely that the eventual disappearance of the penis will lead to the death of the sufferer. Some observers have preferred to use the term 'genital retraction syndrome', under which would be subsumed 'the various cultural specific manifestations; *koro* in the Indonesian archipelago ... *suoyang* among [the] Chinese; *rok joo* in Thailand ... [and] ... *jinginia* in India'.[39] In jinginia, the condition appears to be closely associated with a firm belief that sperm may be leaking from the body into the urine. In the Indian culture there appears to be a strong belief that any form of body wastage of precious fluids is a cause for much concern (see also Chapter five). In Chinese culture, which is said to have been much preoccupied with anxiety over sexual excess, such preoccupation finds expression in the ancient belief concerning the need to keep a balance between *yin* and *yang* elements (female and male representations of important life forces). It is believed that as a result of intercourse (particularly if of a promiscuous nature), and as a result of nocturnal emissions, there may be an unbalanced loss of yang elements. It has also been observed, particularly in early times, that there was much overt expression of disapproval of illicit sexual relationships; the literature is full of serious warnings about the physical ills that may result from these.

Chinese culture has also supported a considerable emphasis upon the importance of spermatic fluids and the threat to life that may ensue if loss of them occurs. Even in more modern times it has been known for children to be threatened with severe penalties for misdemeanours in relation to micturition habits. Numerous ancient Chinese medical writings refer to retraction of the penis into the abdomen (this was probably associated with what would be described today as peritonitis accompanied by oedema) and such texts refer to the likelihood of loss of life occurring. Texts concerning fitness also emphasised the need for sportsmen and boxers to develop their bodies to the point where they could resist kicks and blows, especially to the genital area. Such blows were regarded as having a fatal potentiality. In particular a kick known as *Liau Yin Tui* aimed at the genitals was regarded as a lethal form of attack. This Chinese cultural backcloth to genitality appears to have been drawn upon by David Henry Hwang in his very successful play *M Butterfly*. In this drama, which is a blend of erotic phantasy, history, espionage, and politics, the author depicts the manner in which a diplomat sustains a twenty-year relationship with a woman only to find that his 'mistress' has, in fact, been a man. The play has strong suggestions of ambivalent attitudes towards the expression of sexuality and these pervade the drama powerfully. In a more general context, it is of interest to note the account of one observer who reports upon the 'pre-operative transsexual who was performing as a topless female dancer, who told ... [him] ... that one way to disguise the male genitalia was to push the penis inside the body, tape over it and push the scrotum between the legs'.[40]

In addition to these illustrations from eastern countries, it is important to note that examples have also been reported in western communities; these have included the United States, Canada, and Sweden. The phenomenon has also been observed in Israel and Nigeria. As already briefly noted, the belief is usually accompanied by a degree of anxiety amounting to panic, sweating, nausea, and palpitations. Some observers have suggested that when seen in western communities it is best regarded as an acute reaction to a variety of stresses. In such instances it has been seen as a symptom associated with other psychiatric and physical disorders. Examples described in the literature include the major psychoses, alcoholic hepatitis,[41] epilepsy and other neurological disorders,[42] syphilis, urinary disorders, vitamin deficiency, and herniae. When manifested in western countries some authorities take the view that only a partial presentation of the classical form of the syndrome is being seen and that such presentation is rather different from that described in some of the earlier literature.[43]

Some illustrations

The beliefs and practices described above seem to find expression in some of the cases reported upon by a wide range of clinical and anthropological observers. One such observer describes (in greater detail than that reported upon here) a fairly typical presentation of the condition. This concerned the case of a 32-year-old Chinese cook who suffered from great fears of penile retraction. His family background was disturbed and he suffered very considerable guilt about his long-standing indulgence in sexual promiscuity; however, his guilt about the latter was not sufficient to ensure its cessation. To achieve relief of his symptoms he adopted all manner of indigenous remedies. These included drinking his own urine, that of others, and taking various herbal remedies. When he found his penis shrinking into his abdomen he

> would become very anxious and hold on to his penis in terror.
> Holding his penis, he would faint, with severe vertigo and
> pounding of his heart ... at night he would find that his penis had
> shrunk to a length of only one centimetre and he would pull it
> out and then he would be able to relax and go to sleep.[44]

He had a considerable fear of nocturnal emissions as he would lose *chih* (vital body essence). The means that this sufferer took to prevent retraction would appear to be modest in comparison with other measures reported in the literature. These have included specially devised hooks, clamps, weights, and splints of various kinds in order to prevent the organ's disappearance.[45] The use of such implements would often cause a degree of genital damage which then required surgical intervention. One can only speculate as to whether such draconian activity on the part of the sufferer was also undertaken as a means of further punishment in order to assuage guilt over their real or imagined sexual misdemeanours. The overall picture one has of such sufferers is that they are usually youngish males, shy, introverted, anxious, with highly impressionable personalities. Therefore they are likely to be more than averagely fearful and perhaps ambivalent about sexual behaviour and the real or imagined disorders that may be associated with its over-indulgence. A long-standing preoccupation with the size of the penis is not an uncommon feature in some of these cases. Such preoccupations may well lead to comparisons being made with those believed to be better endowed. The preoccupation is not uncommon in many cultures and is a well-known pastime amongst early adolescent schoolboys. However, in cultures which place a premium upon modesty and reticence about sexuality it may be that this encourages a belief in the value of small and unobtrusive male sexual organs. In this way a conflict situation may be set up on some young males as they develop sexually. This may well lead to guilt and a preoccupation with the physical expression of sex. The fact that culture and social environment can play a significant part in the manifestation of such phenomena is well attested to in the occasional reports of koro 'epidemics'. Rubin summarises the essential features of the epidemic in Singapore in 1967. During a ten-day period, 469 cases were reported. These cases appear to have occurred after it had been reported that people who had eaten the meat of pigs that had been innoculated with anti-swine fever vaccine would develop sexual changes. Rumours abounded that such meat was not wholesome and could cause koro and that this might possibly be lethal. The number of reported cases grew dramatically. Public education via the media emphasised that the meat was harmless and that koro was not due to any physical cause but to fear. Following such publicity the epidemic waned quickly without recurrence.[46] It is also of interest that in this outbreak 5 per cent of the sufferers were women. Koro-type symptoms are not common in females; when they do occur, they appear as a particular anxiety about shrinking of the nipples or vulva.

Management

In cases where koro-like symptoms are associated with overt psychiatric illness, treatment of the latter is likely to bring about improvement in the overall condition of the patient and an accompanying improvement of the koro-type phenomena. It is not at all easy to find clear indications as to where koro should fit into current psychiatric classifications. The third (revised) edition of the *Diagnostic and Statistical Manual of Mental Disorders* would seem to make provision for the condition to be included under any of the following classifications: either 300.01 Panic Disorders without Agoraphobia; or 300.70 Undifferentiated Somatoform Disorders or 302.90 Other Sexual Disorders.[47] In cases where the cultural background appears to have played a prominent part it would seem from most reports that counselling about sexual matters and attempts to allay feelings of guilt and anxiety afford fairly speedy resolution of the problem.

Summary

An examination of the various studies that have been made would seem to demonstrate that culture plays a very prominent part in lending colour (moulding) to the phenomenon of koro-type behaviours, but it is not by any means conclusively causal.[48] The term 'genital retraction syndrome' is probably to be preferred. Under this description can be subsumed the cultural variants and different postulated causes. Three possible manifestations have been suggested using this rubric.

> Those who experience a true physiological reaction (a possible reaction that seems to have been somewhat neglected by many workers) .... Those who experience panic fear of genital retraction in response to real or imagined environmental insult; the chronic somatizers who portray culturally patterned illnesses.[49] (By somatization is meant the presentation of personal and social unease through physical complaints and a means of authenticating the search for medical help.)

In my view this form of differentiation can not only aid diagnosis and management, but serves to encourage clearer thinking about a puzzling and unusual phenomenon.

Some other syndromes

In concluding this chapter brief reference will be made to four other so-called culture-bound syndromes.[50] These would appear to be very heavily culturally determined; there are also widely divergent views as to whether they are even manifestations of actual illness, and, even if they are, what kind of illnesses they represent.

Susto

Susto (Espanto) is found predominantly in Latin-American communities where it is seen as an anxiety syndrome characterised by insomnia, phobias, reduction of sex drive, trembling, palpitations, vomiting, and other features of anxiety states. The belief exists in some areas that if the 'fright' reaches a vital organ such as the heart then death will ensue. The disorder appears to be based upon a complex mixture of beliefs which are concerned with the ways in which the balance of the body may be upset by supernatural means. (Cf. the discussion on p. 53 of *yin* and *yang* forces in relation to koro.) Whatever the strength of such 'superstitious' beliefs, observers have noted that they share 'with modern theories of abnormal behaviour the notion of environmental stress; of the patient's vulnerability to illness or misfortune, which may be brought about by the patient's own behaviour in relation to cultural norms; and of illness as a reflection of the alteration of something *vital* within the individual' (emphasis added).[51]

Latah

This is often described as an hysterical-type reaction, seen predominantly in middle-aged females in lower socio-economic and less well-educated groups. It is known by a wide variety of other names, such as *Arctic hysteria, miryachit* or *olonism* in Russia. In Mongolia, it is known as *belenci*, and in northern Japan as *imu*. The syndrome seems to have as one of its key features a reaction to sudden stress which takes the form of a sudden fright or 'start'.[52] Such an occurrence may result in a variety of reactions such as uncontrollable laughing, the utterance of obscenities, and the repetition of words and behaviour of others. Between episodes the individual may behave quite normally. The explosiveness and violence of the outburst have much in common with some of the amok-like states already described; and a number of the features are similar to those seen in some states of possession (see Chapter three). The expression of symptoms seems to be determined very much by prevailing cultural norms. Because of this, some observers regard it as a 'state' rather than as a disease.

Windigo/Wihtigo/Whitico/Wihtiko

Brief reference was made to this phenomenon in Chapter three. As we have seen, its key characteristic appears to be a compulsive desire to eat human flesh whilst under the delusion that one is possessed by a supernatural being (Windigo). There are reports of it having been observed amongst various North-American Indian groups such as the Algonkians, the Cree, the Salteaux, and the Ojibwa. Such manifestations as have been reported upon seem to occur most in areas of great privation and hunger in which depressive reactions may be quite likely, accompanied by delusional beliefs. It would certainly seem very difficult to classify it clearly within any western psychiatric typologies since it has features of hysteria, depression, and syndromes related to sensory deprivation disorder.[53] It could be seen as having tenuous links with other manifestations of human flesh consumption as in vampirism and necrophagia (see Chapter five).

Pibloktoq (Piblokto)

This phenomenon has been found predominantly among Greenland Eskimo females. It is characterised by a woman singing or swaying rhythmically, then tearing off her clothes and running in the snow or throwing herself into icy water. This behaviour may be accompanied by breast beating, hand clapping, and mimicry of the sounds of birds and/or other animals. This frenetic activity will normally be followed by a state of collapse. Upon recovery the subject will awake in a state of clear consciousness and then resume normal activity. Various explanations have been proffered. It has been described as a form of Arctic hysteria, as a rare epileptic phenomenon, and as a result of some other organic malfunction. Some observers have suggested multiple causation in a setting exacerbated by adverse climatic conditions.[54]

Summary

These four syndromes would seem to have in common sudden or violent reactions to some form of crisis or stress; there would also appear to be hysterical features in all of them. Having said this, it does not take us much further, because in other respects the conditions do not fit comfortably into any western psychiatric classification. It would seem likely that many forms of psychiatric illness may determine the manifestation of these four rare disorders, but the manner in which they are manifested is powerfully determined by culture. Some writers have suggested that, as many of these minority groups in which these states occur become increasingly westernised, the phenomena are likely to diminish and eventually disappear altogether.[55]

Conclusions

It is hoped that in this chapter one key factor will have become clear, namely that the *subjective experience* of illness appears to be culture bound, for culture appears with some consistency to shape and delineate a person's interpretation of, and expressed response to, symptoms.[56] Endeavours to fit such behaviours into neat western-orientated categories are compounded by the difficulties of obtaining adequate and wholly accurate translations of terms used to describe these phenomena in various cultures. In addition, we may not always make sufficient allowance for the reluctance of those being studied to describe intimate and highly emotive thoughts and feelings. For our purposes 'Culture-bound syndromes ... [are best seen] ... as episodic dramatic reactions specific to a particular community, locally identified as discrete patterns of behaviour, and which are consistent over time, located for each generation in a continuing cultural tradition.'[57] Finally, it has been suggested that we in the west may well have our own culture-bound syndromes, 'overdoses, agoraphobia, and some forms of shoplifting and baby snatching are western culture-bound syndromes which articulate both personal predicament and public concerns, usually structural opposition between age-groups and sexes'.[58] The major task, therefore, is to keep our minds (and hearts) open and allow the debate on these fascinating and revealing aspects of human conduct to continue.

Notes and references

1. See L. Marano, '*Windigo* Psychosis: The Anatomy of an Emic-Etic Confusion', in R.C. Simons and C.C. Hughes (eds), *The Culture-bound Syndromes: Folk Illnesses of Psychiatric and Anthropological Interest*, Lancaster, D. Reidel, 1985, pp. 411–448.
2. One such, in the U.K., is R. Littlewood. See, for example, his 'Russian Dolls and Chinese Boxes: An Anthropological Approach to the Implicit Models of Comparative Psychiatry', in J.L. Cox (ed.), *Transcultural Psychiatry*, London, Croom Helm, 1986, Chapter 4.
3. See, for example, J.E. Carr, 'Ethno-behaviourism and the Culture-bound Syndromes', in Simons and Hughes, op. cit., pp. 199–224.
4. M.G. Kenny, 'Paradox Lost: The Latah Problem Revisited', in Simons and Hughes, op. cit., p. 66. Kenny seems to take the view that amok is highly specific to the Malay part of the world and that its genesis pertains to specific concepts of masculine honour.
5. P. Rack, *Race, Culture and Mental Disorder*, London, Tavistock, 1982, p. 148.

6. A. Kiev, *Transcultural Psychiatry*, Harmondsworth, Penguin Books, 1972, p. 78.
7. L. Appleby and S. Wesseley, 'Public Attitudes to Mental Illness: The Influence of the Hungerford Massacre', *Medicine, Science and the Law*, 1988, vol. 28, pp. 291–295.
8. M. Menuck, 'Clinical Assessment of Dangerous Behaviour', in M.H. Ben-Aron, S.J. Hucker and C.D. Webster (eds), *Clinical Criminology: The Assessment and Treatment of Criminal Behaviour*, Clarke Institute of Psychiatry, University of Toronto, Canada, 1985, p. 30. See also H. Merskey, *The Analysis of Hysteria*, London, Ballière Tindall, 1979.
9. H.B.M. Murphy, 'The Historical Development of Transcultural Psychiatry', in Cox, op. cit., Chapter 2.
10. J. Westermeyer, 'Amok', in C.T.H. Friedmann and R.A. Faguet (eds), *Extraordinary Disorders of Human Behaviour*, London, Plenum Press, 1982, Chapter 10.
11. B.G. Burton-Bradley, 'The Hungerford Massacre and its Aftermath', *British Journal of Psychiatry*, 1987, vol. 151, Letter, p. 866.
12. Kiev, op. cit., p. 102.
13. Westermeyer, op. cit., p. 182.
14. A. Kleinman, 'Anthropology and Psychiatry: The Role of Culture in Cross-cultural Research on Illness', *British Journal of Psychiatry*, 1987, vol. 151, pp. 447–454.
15. Kleinman, op. cit., p. 453.
16. Kleinman, ibid.
17. Carr, op. cit., p. 203
18. G. Devereux, 'Normal and Abnormal: The Key Problem of Psychiatric Anthropology', in J.B. Casagrande and T. Gladwin (eds), *Some Uses of Anthropology: Theoretical and Applied*, Anthropological Society of Washington, U.S.A., 1956, pp. 3–48 (quoted in Kiev, op. cit., p. 105).
19. Westermeyer, op. cit. See also his chapter 'Sudden Mass Assault with Grenade: An Epidemic Form from Laos', in Simons and Hughes, op. cit., pp. 225–235. Carr (op. cit.) also describes it as 'Sudden Mass Assault Taxon'. This includes the Malaysian form of amok and similar instances of world-wide indiscriminate homicide.
20. R.J. Wilkinson, *Papers on Malay Subjects, Part III*, 1925 (pp. 5–6), Federated Malay States Government Press, Kuala Lumpur. Quoted in Carr, op. cit., p. 212.
21. B.G. Burton-Bradley, 'The Amok Syndrome in Papua and New Guinea', in Simons and Hughes, op. cit., pp. 237–249.
22. B.G. Burton-Bradley, op. cit., p. 243.
23. B.G. Burton-Bradley, op. cit. 1987. The word 'hypereridism' is attributed to E. Lindemann, see *Epidemiology of Mental Disorder*, New York, Millbank Memorial Fund, 1950.
24. B.G. Burton-Bradley, op. cit. 1987, p. 866.
25. J. Arboleda-Florez, 'Amok', in Simons and Hughes, op. cit., pp. 251–262.
26. See *Diagnostic and Statistical Manual of Mental Disorders* (3rd edn revised), American Psychiatric Association, Washington D.C., 1980,

298:80 and 312:315. The classification does not appear in the Revised Edition (*DSM III [R]*) 1987. The problems of trying to match so-called culture-bound syndromes to current psychiatric classifications is usefully discussed by Kroll. See J. Kroll, 'Cross-cultural Psychiatry, Culture-bound Syndromes and DSM III', *Current Opinion in Psychiatry*, 1988, vol. 1, pp. 46–52.

27. The extracts and references are from the *Independent*, 20 August 1987, 21 August 1987, 26 August 1987, 30 September 1987 and 1 October 1987.
28. *Independent*, 26 September 1987.
29. *Independent*, 26 September 1987.
30. *Independent*, 29 October 1988.
31. *Independent*, 29 October 1988.
32. *Independent*, 29 October 1988.
33. *Independent*, 1 May 1989 and 2 May 1989. At the time of writing Sartin is said to be too mentally ill to be produced in court. An apparently comparable case is that of the Frenchman Dornier, who killed 14 people on 12 July 1989, *Independent*, 13 July 1989. A more recent Canadian case is that of Marc Lepine, aged 25, an Algerian-Canadian. He killed 14 students at Montreal University and then killed himself. He was said to have been 'always frustrated with women', became preoccupied with the manner in which they had treated him badly and was determined to take his revenge. He appeared to have been a loner, from a broken home, and obsessed with war films. He had no prior criminal or psychiatric history as far as can be ascertained. He bought the gun without any difficulty and the gun shop assistant is alleged to have said, 'He didn't appear any crazier than anyone else actually, he was a bit of a joker.' *Independent*, 9 December 1989.
34. In relation to schizophrenia see N.L. Gittelson and S. Levine, 'Subjective Ideas of Sexual Change in Male Schizophrenics', *British Journal of Psychiatry*, 1966, vol. 112, pp. 1171–1173.
35. J. Kroll, op. cit. For a short account of views on self-perception and depersonalisation see C.S. Mellor, 'Depersonalisation and Self-perception', in *The Psychopathology of Body Image* (eds K.J.B. Rix and R.P. Snaith), *British Journal of Psychiatry* (Supplement No. 2), 1988, vol. 153, pp. 15–19.
36. A number of authors have explored the history and derivation of the term. See, for example, G.S. Devan and S. Hong, 'Koro and Schizophrenia in Singapore', *British Journal of Psychiatry*, 1987, vol. 150, pp. 106–107; P.M. Yap, 'Koro – A Culture-bound Depersonalisation Syndrome', *British Journal of Psychiatry*, 1965, vol. 111, pp. 43–50; R.T. Rubin, 'Koro (Shook Yang): A Culture-bound Psychogenic Syndrome', in Friedmann and Faguet, op. cit., Chapter 9; J.W. Edwards, 'Indigenous Koro – A Genital Syndrome of Insular Southeast Asia: A Critical Review', in Simon and Hughes, op. cit., pp. 169–191.
37. A.L. Gwee (Gwee Ah Leng), 'Koro – A Cultural Disease', in Simons and Hughes, op. cit., pp. 155–159.

38. A.L. Gwee (Gwee Ah Leng), 'Koro – A Cultural Disease', *Singapore Medical Journal*, 1963, vol. 4, pp. 119–122.
39. Edwards, op. cit., p. 184.
40. Edwards, op. cit., p. 187.
41. See, for example, T.H. Holden, 'Koro Syndrome Associated with Alcohol Induced Systemic Disease in a Zulu', *British Journal of Psychiatry*, 1987, vol. 151, pp. 685–697.
42. See also R. Durst and P. Rosca-Rebaudengo, 'Koro Secondary to a Tumour in the Corpus Callosum', *British Journal of Psychiatry*, 1988, vol. 153, pp. 251–254.
43. See G.E. Berrios and S.J. Morley, 'Koro-like Symptoms in a non-Chinese Subject', *British Journal of Psychiatry*, 1984, vol. 145, pp. 331–334.
44. Kiev, op. cit., pp. 79–82.
45. For a fuller description and photographs see Rubin in Friedmann and Faguet, op. cit., pp. 158–163.
46. Rubin in Friedmann and Faguet, op. cit., pp. 164–167.
47. American Psychiatric Association, op. cit.
48. See O.I. Ifabumuyi and G.C. Rwegellern, 'Koro in a Nigerian Male Patient: A Case Report', in Simons and Hughes, op. cit., pp. 161–163.
49. Edwards, op. cit., p. 186.
50. In this section of the chapter I have drawn quite heavily upon work by C.T.H. Friedmann, 'The So-called Hystero-psychoses: Latah, Windigo, and Pibloktoq', in Friedmann and Faguet, op. cit., Chapter 13. See also Kiev, op. cit., Chapter 4. A fuller anthropological treatment may be found in Simons and Hughes, op. cit., particularly pp. 41–113.
51. Kiev, op. cit., pp. 83–84. For more detailed discussion see A.J. Rubel, C.W.O. Nell and R. Collado, 'The Folk-illness called *Susto*', in Simons and Hughes, op. cit., pp. 333–350.
52. Simons and Hughes in their development of a taxonomy for so-called culture-bound disorders refer to it in the context of a 'startle-matching taxon'. See Simons and Hughes, op. cit., *Section A* and *especially* commentary by Hughes at pp. 111–113.
53. See Marano in Simons and Hughes, op. cit., pp. 411–448 for a very comprehensive anthropological account of this curious phenomenon.
54. For a very interesting anthropo-psychiatric account see Z. Gussow, '*Pibloktoq* (Hysteria) Among the Polar Eskimo: An Ethnopsychiatric Study', in Simons and Hughes, op. cit., pp. 271–287.
55. See Friedmann, in Friedmann and Faguet, op. cit., p. 227.
56. R. Angel and P. Thoits, 'The Impact of Culture on the Cognitive Structures of Illness', *Culture, Medicine and Psychiatry*, 1987, vol. 11, pp. 465–484.
57. M. Lipsedge, 'Cultural Influences on Psychiatry', *Current Opinion in Psychiatry*, 1989, vol. 2, pp. 267–272.
58. R. Littlewood and M. Lipsedge, 'The Butterfly and the Serpent: Culture, Psychopathology and Bio-medicine', *Culture, Medicine and Psychiatry*, 1987, vol. 11, pp. 289–336.

Chapter five

Blood relations: unusual encounters with death and the dead

'There are more things in heaven and earth, Horatio,
Than are dreamt of in your philosophy.'
(*Hamlet*, Act I, Scene v)

'Because there are innumerable things beyond the range of
human understanding, we constantly use symbolic terms to
represent concepts that we cannot define or fully comprehend.'
(Carl Jung, On the Nature of the Psyche,
Collected Works, volume 8)

The subject matter of this chapter, the longest in this small book, illustrates more clearly than any of the others the need for the multi-disciplinary approach referred to earlier. In order to enrich our understanding we must explore the territories of anthropology, folk-lore, mythology, art, and theology as well as those disciplines that concern themselves more specifically with seriously abnormal behaviour such as abnormal psychology, psychiatry, forensic medicine, toxicology, and pathology. The major part of this chapter is devoted to a study of vampirism since it seems to illustrate quite graphically the need for multi-disciplinary study. I shall also consider certain other topics which seem to fit reasonably well into the context of this chapter, though it *could* be argued that their inclusion is a little arbitrary. These include lycanthropy, zombiism, necrophilia, and certain other practices which link sexuality with death.

The vampire as paradigm

My interest in this particular topic was first aroused by an account by two doctors working in South Africa of what they described as 'a presentation of three cases of clinical vampirism and a re-evaluation of Haigh, the "acid-bath" murderer'.[1] In respect of Haigh's case, the authors of the article seemed to me to be somewhat mistaken in their belief in describing his activities as vampiristic.[2] As is well known, Haigh attempted to simulate insanity; part of this simulation was a claim to have drunk the blood of his victims. A very useful account of Haigh's trial for murder and the psychiatric evidence pertaining to it may be found in Neustatter's book *The Mind of the Murderer*.[3] Because of my long-standing interest in strange behaviour, and in the borderline between 'madness' and 'badness', I considered it worthwhile to examine this apparently rare and little written about phenomenon more closely. In order to do so, I circulated a letter of enquiry to some forty-five psychiatrists and others of my acquaintance in an effort to ascertain whether they had come across vampiristic phenomena in their clinical work. A brief analysis of the composition of my respondents is given in Table 5.1.

Table 5.1[a] Respondents

Psychiatrists	34[b]
Anthropologists	5
Ministers of religion	1
Clinical psychologists	1
Pathologists	1[c]
Others	3

Notes:

[a] The data were collected during the period May 1983 – February 1984. Since the publication of the paper in October 1984, I have received a steady flow of correspondence and requests for further information. There is obviously a great deal of current interest in the topic.[4]

[b] A further six did not reply to my enquiry. Of the 34 who did, 18 were either forensic psychiatrists (three being professors) or had extensive experience in examining and treating deviants and offenders. The group also included the medical directors of Broadmoor, Park Lane, and Rampton Special Hospitals. Several correspondents were kind enough to send more than one communication as and when they came across further material. A number also consulted other colleagues before replying; thus the data collected came from considerably more than my 34 respondents.

[c] A professor of pathology with very extensive experience of forensic work; he had consulted several colleagues before replying.

The sample and some inferences

The sample of respondents is, of course, highly selective because it consisted of psychiatrists and colleagues well known to me who would be likely to have an interest in the topic (notably either forensic psychiatrists or those general psychiatrists known to me to have a specific interest in seriously abnormal conduct). However, as is so often the case, what began as a very modest and small-scale enquiry 'mushroomed'. As already indicated, my original group of psychiatric respondents suggested other colleagues and fellow workers who might be helpful. It was possible, therefore, to obtain data not only from those in the psychiatric field, but from anthropologists and others in this country and abroad. However, it is important to stress that the number of respondents is very small and great care should be taken in interpreting the clinical data referred to later. In addition, the material from folk-lore and mythology surrounding body fluids (particularly blood) is not only ubiquitous, but extremely complex and voluminous. Only a fraction of it is dealt with here. Some of the references cited should be consulted by those who wish to study this fascinating topic further.

The significance of blood and other body substances

The mystical and powerful properties of blood and other body substances are well attested to in the ancestral recesses of recorded human experience. Before we consider briefly the significance and ubiquity of blood ritual and observance, it is useful to note that blood is but one of a variety of body substances held to be endowed with special (scatatherapeutic) powers. In addition to blood, excreta, urine and semen (both human and other animal) feature extensively in the literature of mythology and folk-lore. For example, urine has been used for centuries in various parts of the world for the treatment of such diverse complaints as chilblains, toothache, and impotence.[5] The biblical statement that 'he that believeth in me as the Scripture hath said, out of his belly shall flow rivers of living water' (*John* 7:38) has often been cited in support of such beliefs. In similar fashion, human excrement was widely used in medicinal treatments.[6] Seminal fluid was also considered to have very important properties. That derived from animals (notably bulls) was widely sought after and used for the purpose of inducing and ensuring human virility. Folk-lore has it that 'fresh human semen was ... largely sought by vampires'.[7] It is also on record that semen collected at the point of ejaculation by a man at the moment of death by hanging was said to be a particularly powerful scatatherapeutic agent. If it was not collected, as was frequently the case, and it fell to the ground, it was said to generate the mandrake, a plant frequently used in demonological rites.[8] There is little doubt that superstition and fear play a prominent part in the background to our attitudes to many so-called modern social and medical problems. The phenomena of venereal disease, of HIV infection, and of AIDS are good examples. Venereal disease is now a treatable condition and is no longer such a symbol of guilt and of mortality, yet fear and superstition still surround it. AIDS is, as yet, untreatable and emotions surrounding it are powerful. Paul Barker makes a comparison between the death of Count Dracula in Bram Stoker's novel and the manner in which, some ninety years later, a young man suffering from AIDS died in hospital.

His parents were not allowed to see his body; it was placed into two sealed bags, one inside the other and was buried in a special steel coffin. Heavy flagstones were placed above his burial place. In the same article Barker reminds us how Ibsen's *Ghosts* – a play about syphilis – caused such a fierce outcry when it was first produced. Barker is making the important point that 'You cannot detach present-day reactions from how people felt about such insidious threats in the past.'[9]

The specific significance of blood

In his book *The Gift Relationship*, Titmuss points out that 'there is a bond that links all men and women in the world so closely and intimately that every difference of colour, religious belief and cultural heritage is insignificant beside it'.[10] He also stressed that the 'history of every people assigns to blood a unique importance'.[11] It seems to bear a close parallel to the powerful and unique phenomenon of fire.[12] Blood rituals and beliefs abound; power has always been associated with its possession and consumption. It is noteworthy for our purposes that its loss has been associated with impotence, ill-fate, and tragedy.[13] However, its loss by deliberate intervention such as blood-letting is also well known. Evidence of mediaeval blood-letting on a grand scale has emerged following an archaeological excavation near Edinburgh. Chemical analysis has shown that a monastic hospital was used as a 'dump' for human blood. The rules of the order required that all monks be bled to the point of unconsciousness between 'seven and 12 times a year'! It was held that loss of blood helped to create a balance between what they held to be the four main aspects of human temperament – pessimism, optimism, anger, and apathy.[14] This would appear to be similar to the balancing of *yang* and *yin* forces outlined in our observations on koro in Chapter four. An anthropological approach to the subject matter emphasises that blood rites and rituals must be seen in a broad situational context. It is important to stress the difference between an *individual* piece of behaviour (for example, blood-sucking or ingestion) and that which is sanctioned as a culturally recognised institution – be it approved or deviant. Such relationships, as we noted in Chapter four, are extremely complex. The work of Lévi-Strauss and his followers has done much to try to elucidate the complex nature of these relationships and the variations in customs, myths, and the patterns of these manifold institutional beliefs in a wide range of cultures.[15] In some of these, blood ingestion may have been necessary for dietary or immunological purposes; in others, blood ingestion forms a part of cannibalistic rites and practices.[16] In

Madagascar, for example, the dead are removed from their burial places in the ceremony of *famadihana*. This ceremony is designed to enable the dead to give to the living the meaning of life.

> In the open, the shroud is removed from the corpse. Those seeking a blessing and happiness dip their hands in the decomposed matter and eat it or smear it on their faces. After the remains have been carefully re-wrapped in new material, the women of the immediate family sit together in a line. The cocoon-like parcels are placed on their laps as they pray for fertility and are then put on their shoulders as they pray for happiness. They seek ancestral blessings in a kind of dance of the dead.[17]

In some parts of the world in acute survival situations it is, of course, not uncommon for blood and flesh to be consumed as a means of survival, as, for example, in cases of shipwreck and abandonment. In many cultures it was customary to ingest the blood of those defeated in battle in order to gain strength for battles to come. The Cretans were said to fertilise 'Mother Earth' with the blood of their victims. It is reported by one authority that such blood rituals were especially important in the Balkan countries. 'Thus one group of Balkan pirates displayed the mutilated corpse of the Holy Roman Emperor's envoy in a church. Wives then demonstrated solidarity with their husbands by licking the bloody body.'[18] In some Greek villages, it is not uncommon to threaten an enemy with violent death by saying 'I shall drink your blood.'[19] Also, there would appear to be links with the ritual partaking of wine as a substitute for blood in religious ceremonial, the incorporation of which is seen as strong and life-enhancing. The *Book of Leviticus* also reminds us that blood rituals were used not only for purposes of atonement but also for the purification of priests (8: 23). In one clinical contribution the authors quote a patient's citation of Scripture in support of his alleged cannibalistic and vampiristic activities.[20] The relevant biblical text is of interest: 'Whoso eateth my flesh, and drinketh my blood, hath eternal life; and I will raise him up at the last day ...' (*John* 6: 54); 'For my flesh is meat indeed and my blood is drink indeed' (6: 55); 'Except ye eat the flesh of the son of man, and drink his blood, ye hath no life in you' (6: 53). In a footnote the authors of the paper go on to make the important point that 'the religious benefit spiritually, not corporally from Communion'.[21] The metaphor, however, is a powerful one; even those who are not of the Christian faith cannot fail to be moved by the powerful imagery of the rite of Communion, its preparation, and the manner in which the officiant concludes the ritual. Even more powerful images of the association between blood and Christian worship are afforded in some of the world's great paintings. Perhaps one of the most moving and graphic depictions of this association is the painting of the Crucifixion by Nardo Di Cione (*c*. 1300–1365). In this we see the figure of Christ with the blood from the palms of His hands and from the wound in His side being collected into vessels held by angels. The blood from His feet runs down to a skull lying on the ground at the foot of the crucifixion stake. Powerful imagery indeed.

Other traditions reveal a decided degree of ambivalence about the use of, or contact with, blood. In some cultures, menstrual blood has been highly prized for its life-giving and other potent properties, particularly that coming from a virgin on her first day's flow. In others, such as in Papua New Guinea, the ritual of nasal mutilation and bleeding in males is said to serve a similar purpose to that of female menstruation and is a much valued phenomenon.[22] It is an interesting matter for speculation whether the alleged 'proving' activities of some groups of so-called 'Hell's Angels', as illustrated in their sometimes seeking intercourse with menstruating women, have their origins in similar ancient beliefs, rather than purely being acts of aggression and repugnant defilement. Contrary views also prevail – as in the Orthodox Jewish belief which prohibits all physical and sexual contacts with a menstruating woman. Biblical authority requires that the woman should take a ritual cleansing bath (The 'Mikvah': *Leviticus* 15: 49) following the cessation of her menstrual flow.[23] It is also of interest to note that Orthodox Jews will eat meat only if it is Kosher, i.e. that killed in a manner that removes all traces of blood (*Leviticus* 17: 10–16). These brief background comments should suffice to place the rest of this chapter in perspective.

The vampire myth – the unquiet dead

The phenomenon of the vampire is both powerful and world-wide. It is often thought to be of purely Slavic origin, but in fact, its ancestry may be traced back to the very earliest civilisations. There appear to be two major notions underlying the myth. First, that a malign spirit can take over a corpse and use it for its own nefarious activities. Second, that the soul of an individual considered to be too evil to be allowed into the world of the dead can continue to inhabit his or her body in the form of a vampire – the great 'undead' (or revenants). The term appears to have been applied to blood-sucking ghosts and then to blood-sucking bats. In many accounts of the development of the phenomenon, the vampire is usually taken to be a dead person who has returned in spirit from the grave for the purpose of destroying and sucking the blood of living persons.[24] The anthropologist Du Bulay has summarised very usefully much material concerning types of vampire. She lists nine types:[25]

1. Those who did not receive the full and due rites of burial.
2. Those who met with sudden and violent death (including suicide) or who had been the victims of vendetta type activities and whose deaths had been unavenged.
3. Stillborn children.
4. Those who died under a curse, especially those who perjured themselves through taking God's name in vain.
5. Those who died under the ban of the church – the excommunicate – an important group.
6. Those who died unbaptized or apostate (having abandoned faith).
7. Men of immoral or evil life – particularly those who had dealt in the black arts.
8. Those who had eaten the flesh of a sheep which had been killed by a wolf. (It is interesting how frequently the wolf figures in the folk-lore of vampirism – indeed the phenomenon has given rise to a sub-speciality – lycanthropy – see pp. 80–3.)
9. Those over whose dead bodies a cat or other animal has passed. The reference to a cat in early civilisations such as Greece is of interest because cats appear to figure extensively in the later folk-lore of witchcraft and demonology. It probably also accounts for the ancient custom seen in this country whereby animals are kept away from corpses awaiting burial.[26]

The term

The word 'vampire' has been the subject of various attempts at derivation. In Greek the generic term is *Vrylolakos*. Its more recent derivation can be found in the Turkish word *Uber* or witch, then through the Russian *Upyr*, Magyar, *vampir* or Bulgarian *upir*. The word vampire (occasionally spelt vampyre) appears to have first made its appearance in English writing about the middle of the eighteenth century. Also, in more recent times, it has come to represent greedy or rapacious individuals, more particularly irresistible lovers (mostly female) who may, metaphorically speaking, exsanguinate their victims to the point of death. The fictional vampire bears little relation to his or her folk-loric counterpart but, as we shall see, there are certain aspects that are relevant to the clinical manifestation of the condition.

According to tradition, vampires are corpses, neither dead nor alive – the so-called 'undead'. We probably owe the most detailed explorations of the myth to the late (Reverend) Montague Summers.[27] However, caution is necessary in interpreting the significance of Summers' work. He had been a cleric who converted from the Anglican Church to Roman Catholicism. He certainly seems to have believed not only in a personal devil but in the actual existence of vampires.

> Cases of vampirism may be said to be in our time a rare occult phenomenon. Yet whether we are justified in supposing that they are less frequent today than in past centuries I am far from certain. One thing is plain: not that they do not occur but that they are carefully hushed up and stifled.[28]

Little is known of the true facts of this somewhat enigmatic, unusual but learned man's life. (It is said that all his personal papers simply disappeared immediately after his death.) However, his autobiography, published some thirty years after his death, gives some glimpses that help to put him and his work into perspective as a student of demonology, the occult, and the bizarre.[29] His belief in a personal devil appears to endow much of his writing with a considerable degree of dogma and fervour. Because of this he seemed to show 'no hesitation in taking at face value whatever [had] been documented in folk tales of these "terrible phenomena". The central ambivalence of Summers' analysis, and not a small part of its attraction, is, it seems to me, the way this credulity is supported by an impressive structure of scholarship and observation.'[30] For Summers, the concept of vampirism certainly had evil, sexual, and Satanic connotations:

> The power of the dead to inflict injury upon the living is not merely confined to any ghostly affrightment, but strikes something deeper. The dead may come back in their bodies as malignant monsters eager to carry off the living to the shadowy realm where they have gone before.[31]

As one of my respondents so graphically put it: 'Those who have been properly sent on their way ... i.e. properly shriven and buried ... will arrive at their destination.'[32] For those not so blessed, for example, suicides and others, history shows that a quiet release and transit from this world were not to be theirs – hence the long-standing reluctance to bury suicides in hallowed ground and the need to impale their corpses with stakes through their hearts. The vampire also needed a second burial and the additional rituals of staking, severing the head, and/or burning it. If it was not burned, a clove of garlic might be placed in the mouth.

The vampire in literature

For most people, the phenomenon of the vampire has been best understood, if somewhat erroneously, through the pages of Bram Stoker's classic Gothic novel first published in 1897. To be fair, Stoker did a fair amount of historical research in the British Museum Library in order to obtain what he regarded as authentic background for his novel. It is likely that he based his Count in part upon the malevolent and notorious Vlad the Impaler (1431–1476) or some similar ruler, and in part upon the character of the lesbian murderess Countess Bathory. She is said to have engaged in the black arts and to have drunk the blood of countless young girls after torturing, then murdering, them in order to preserve her own beauty. In point of fact, Stoker's fictional depiction of the Count as a vampire bears little relation to descriptions found in folk-lore. In what is probably the most impressive recent contribution to the study of the vampire phenomenon, Barber shows how the vampires of folk-lore were mostly described as ruddy, bloated, and bucolic looking.[33] A depiction far removed from the image of the thin, somewhat cadaverous, erotic, and sinister aristocratic count. This presentation has, of course, been sustained by the plethora of films on Dracula themes since the 1920s. Actors, such as Bela Lugosi and Christopher Lee, have tended to maintain the original Stoker image. Although Stoker's novel is usually taken to be the first major depiction of the vampire theme, there were a considerable number of novels and other works that embraced vampire themes published before that date. A brief account of some of these may be found in Wilson's introduction and notes to the Oxford University Press edition of *Dracula*, published in 1983 (at pp. vii–xxiii). Some other examples of vampire themes in well-known literary works are Keats' poem *Lamia*, Byron's *The Giaour*, Goethe's *The Bride of Corinth*, Bürger's *Lenore*, Southey's *Thalaba The Destroyer*, Polidori's *The Vampyre*, Gautier's *La Morte Amoureux*, Prest's (or more likely Rymer's) *Varney the Vampyre or the Feast of Blood*, Le Fanu's *Carmilla* and *In a Glass Darkly*, and Maupassant's *The Horla* (an example of psychic vampirism). Other writers who have included vampiric themes in their works are F. Marion Crawford, M.R. James, Conan Doyle, E.P. Benson, and Ray Bradbury. Leatherdale has written a recent and well-documented account of the Dracula novel and the legend.[34] A very recent anthology of vampire stories has been edited by Ryan. This includes tales from 1816 to 1984.[35]

Fostering the legend

Vampire legends in Europe were probably given some factual credibility as a result of inadequate or precipitate burial during times of plague. The plague would of itself have provided added fear in already superstitious times. (We saw in Chapter four how phenomena such as amok and koro could be given heightened credibility in similar fashion.) We may ask therefore what *natural* as distinct from *supernatural* explanations might there be for such phenomena? Barber, in the work already referred to, made an extensive examination of accounts of exhumations of suspected vampires and suggests that forensic pathology holds many of the answers to phenomena thought previously to be of supernatural origin. Such factors as the presence of odd-looking and malnourished vagrants, premature burial, the effects of decomposition, the manner in which decaying corpses change after death and interact with the soil they are buried in, and other post-mortem changes could all help to account for such phenomena. There is little doubt that the stench from putrefaction would give rise to the 'stench of the vampire' – evil being easily associated with noxious odours. Barber sets out certain guidelines for making sense of some of the 'folk-lore':

1. In examining European vampire folklore, ... begin by assuming that few of our informants are deliberately fabricating evidence. Either they are actually observing something or they believe that they are.
2. ... make a sharp distinction between observed phenomena and explanation, for the one may be accurate while the other is not. The explanation will nevertheless often prove helpful to us in determining what the observed phenomena are.
3. When the 'observed phenomena' make no sense to us, we ... try two further hypotheses.
   a. The language of the folkloric account may be metaphorical or inexact because the frame of reference is alien to our own. We must look for the 'core event', peeling back the metaphor until we have something actual. This is less risky than it sounds, because metaphor tends both to be coherent and to reveal its secrets by how it varies from one culture to the next.
   b. ... study the actual phenomena to determine whether it is our informants or we ourselves who lack adequate information.[36]

The porphyria connection

The result of research on the porphyrias has been proffered recently as a further possible explanation of the vampire phenomena.[37] The porphyrias – of which there are a number of variants – are genetic disorders in which the body produces an excess of porphyria which in turn produces excess redness of the eyes, skin and teeth and receding of the upper lip and cracking of the skin. The latter is said to bleed when exposed to light. People who suffer from porphyria fail to produce an enzyme needed by the body to produce haema – the red pigment of blood that is a constitutent of haemoglobin. It has been suggested that in ancient times physicians could only treat such patients by secluding them during the day and by persuading them to drink blood to replace that lost by their bleeding.[38] If this were true, it would serve to enhance the vampire myth. The porphyria theory also has a bearing upon another interesting facet of vampirism – the age-old use of garlic as an *apotropaic* (apotropaics, according to Barber, are methods of turning away evil). A complex series of enzyme reactions takes place when garlic is ingested and this results in the stimulation of haeme. It is thought that, for the person suffering from porphyria, such ingestion would serve to exacerbate the condition and make it more painful. In addition, it has been suggested by one of my correspondents that the pungent odour given off by garlic (due to allyl methyl trisulphide)[39] would also make the sufferer from porphyria try to avoid it at all costs. The porphyria theory has proved popular in recent times, but there is really insufficient evidence to establish a conclusive connection. Perhaps it is best to regard it as just one additional, and quite plausible, theory to bear in mind.

Despite all these possible, and in some cases quite probable, practical explanations, it is quite clear that for a variety of reasons the *myth* has always exerted a firm hold in past and current beliefs and seems likely to continue to do so.[40] Some of these reasons can be summarised at this point as a prelude to a discussion of some clinical aspects of the phenomena: first, the existence of a powerful belief based upon a desire for reunion with dead loved ones; second, the significance of blood as a vital life-giving symbol – in some respects the accounts of vampirism can be seen as a kind of re-affirmation of this symbolic significance, or at least as evidence of a need for it under certain circumstances; third, the phenomenon of blood ingestion as a form of parasitic 'leech-like' activity; fourth, the existence of strong sexual components – notably the vampire's biting 'kiss' as a representation by extension of sadistic, sexual phantasies; fifth, the interesting speculation that the two possibly greatest 'horror' novels ever written – *Frankenstein* and *Dracula* – deal respectively with the

creation of life and with its perpetuation.[41] It may be that this observation helps us to reconcile many of the apparent conflicts concerning
some of the strongest and, for some people, most terrifying of myths; it
illustrates the age-old need to balance the forces of life and death
and, indeed, of good and evil. It will be recalled that I noted the need
for similar 'balancing acts' in earlier chapters of this book.

Clinical aspects

Current prevalence

There appear to be quite well-authenticated accounts of what today
might be regarded as clinical vampiristic behaviour dating from quite
early times.[42] There are also accounts of the allied conditions of necrophagia (eating the flesh of the human dead) and necrophilia (interference with, or sexual molestation of, corpses) and these are the
subject of comment later in this chapter. As one of my respondents
so compellingly put it: it is highly unlikely, even within a well-
established therapeutic relationship, that a patient or offender will
readily divulge information concerning vampiristic or similar activities. This may well account, in part, for the paucity of data and the
fact that few accounts have appeared in the clinical literature.
Although my own original literature survey was a modest one, I have
reason to believe that I garnered most of the relevant papers. Since
the original research was published some additional cases have come
to my attention and these are referred to below. However, even if we
add in these extra case examples, the sum total seems to be very small.
Only two of my respondents (see Table 5.1) could quote accounts
that might be regarded as clinical vampirism (human blood ingestion) in 'pure culture'. One of these was very much a 'third hand'
account and another case was still under investigation. Two of the
three cases cited by Hemphill and his colleague appear to have shown
signs of other disturbance such as long-standing anti-social behaviour and serious chronic delinquency. As mentioned earlier, their
use of Haigh – the 'acid bath murderer' – is somewhat questionable,
since in the first place he appeared to feign insanity and in the second, his story of alleged vampiristic activity seems to have been
entirely uncorroborated. Thirty-three of my psychiatrist respondents
suggested that any vampiristic activities they had come across were
associated with other phenomena and/or psychotic disorder. The
psychiatric conditions that seemed to have the closest associations were,
in order of frequency, schizophreniform disorders, hysteria, severe
personality disorder, and mental retardation. Depression and other
disorders, such as anxiety states or the epilepsies, rarely featured.

Some additional cases

A correspondent, not in my original sample, wrote to me giving details of five cases he had come across, three in a special and two in an ordinary mental hospital. Three of the patients were male and two female. All were thought to be suffering from personality disorder (four of a schizoid or schizo-affective type and one from an atypical bipolar disorder).[43] A further case concerns a young woman who appeared to be suffering from post-puerperal psychosis. She allegedly became convinced that her teeth were growing and that she was turning into a vampire following the birth of her baby. She became so convinced that she might be a danger to the latter that she tied a crucifix around his neck. Although she felt herself to be an acute threat to her baby, she did not in fact harm the child at any time.[44] This example is of interest, since it illustrates the role of a depressive illness in the manifestation of vampiristic feelings. A more graphic case is that of the 19-year-old man who stabbed an elderly widow (the mother of one of his best friends) as a practice run for a 'black-magic' sacrifice. After killing the woman with a kitchen knife he searched out her jugular vein in order to perfect his technique for a ritual killing. It was alleged that the latter was to be performed on a 13-year-old boy to fulfil his ambition to drink human blood and to be granted immortality and eternal youth. He had been obsessed with the occult since he was a small boy and believed implicitly in all the vampire myths and legends. At his trial it was also alleged that he roamed cemeteries at night dressed in a 'Count Dracula' type cape.

At his trial, a psychiatrist said that the defendant had intense urges to bite the necks of adolescent boys and drink their blood because he believed it to have a supernatural quality. He had pleaded not guilty to murder but guilty to manslaughter on the grounds of diminished responsibility. This was accepted and he was sent to a special hospital to be detained without limit of time. It is of interest that none of his close associates had any idea of his bizarre feelings and activities.[45] The interest in the occult is again a notable feature of such cases, as it was in some of the cases of possession described in Chapter four. Two further examples help to illustrate the point. The first concerns a man of 21 who stabbed and killed his flat-mate after an argument. In court it was described as a ritual killing after evidence had been given by the police of black magic regalia and other articles in their flat.[46] The second concerned the case of a man of 24 – a so-called 'devil-worshipper'; he knitted a black woollen doll before killing his 55-year-old homosexual lover with two knives. He is alleged to have told the police 'I felt the devil and his horns on my head when I plunged the knife through his heart.' The court accepted a plea of diminished responsibility and the defendant was ordered to be sent to a special hospital.[47] Occasionally, an individual seems to develop vampiristic tendencies after stimulation from the media. One young man is alleged to have nicked the neck of several of his girl friends in order to satisfy his desire for blood. He is alleged to have told reporters 'It's the actual sucking of the blood that gives me the biggest buzz.' Fortunately, his activities do not appear to have led him into more serious trouble and the newspaper reporting of this particular example borders on the sensational. I quoted it in order to demonstrate the possible influence of the media upon those who may be vulnerable.[48] Such unhealthy trends would *appear* to be on the increase. In East Berlin there are reports of a bizarre East German youth sect, known as Grufties, who occupy themselves by digging up coffins and stealing parts of their contents. Crosses, and funeral sprays, are also taken in order for them to say masses for the dead.[49]

Clinical definition and classification

Some authors suggest that 'compulsive blood taking, uncertain identity and an abnormal interest in death ... are symptoms of the psychopathology of clinical vampirism'.[50] They limit their definition to blood ingestion, whereas others include necrophilic activities. It is important to point out again that vampirism is a useful illustration in which myth, phantasy, and reality converge. Confirmation of such a view comes from some psychoanalytic writing and is of particular relevance because such borderlines have important aetiological and treatment implications.[51] The following classification is derived largely from the material supplied from my respondents and from a synthesis of the literature, in particular a key contribution from Bourguignon.[52] The term vampirism, as already noted, has been used by some to include both necrophagia and necrophilia. It has also been used to cover certain sadistic activities in relation to serious sexual assault, particularly in those cases in which frenzied aggressive sexual activity has taken place. The word has also been used to include self/auto-vampirism. The following is a five-fold classification, modified after Bourguignon.

1. Complete vampirism – involving ingestion of blood, necrophilic activity and necro-sadism. This would include what some have described as haemolagnia (blood lust).[53]
2. Vampirism without ingestion of blood or consumption of dead flesh. Bourguignon describes this as necrophilia and states that it consists of sexual satisfaction derived from touching (interference) or actual intercourse with a cadaver.

(I consider necrophilia as a separate entity on pp. 84–7.)
3. Vampirism without death being involved.[54]
4. Auto-vampirism. This would include those cases in which an individual derives satisfaction from the ingestion of his or her own blood. A sub-division of auto-vampirism can also be made:
   a. Self-induced bleeding with ingestion of blood.
   b. Voluntary bleeding with re-ingestion of blood.
   c. A further sub-classification which would include a condition described as autohaematofetishism (pleasure, mostly sexual, derived from the sight of blood drawn up in a syringe in the process of intravenous drug addictive practice).[55]

A number of my respondents also described patients in which self-mutilation had been linked with minor blood ingestive activity; mostly this was associated with attention-seeking behaviour.[56] In a case reported in the literature, a female patient stored her own blood in order to look at it in times of stress since she felt this activity had a calming effect upon her. One of my respondents described a somewhat similar case in which a male patient stored his blood to achieve a similar result.

Aetiological and treatment considerations

As has been suggested, the literature on clinical vampirism is sparse. The phenomenon seems to manifest itself alongside, or to be part of, other conditions rather than, as some have suggested, existing as a distinct entity. Some of my respondents pointed out that it was not infrequently associated with serious sadistic sexual offending where biting and perhaps blood ingestion were occasionally manifested. It is interesting to speculate to what extent such activity is but a very serious pathological extension of the more normal and ubiquitous phenomenon of the 'love-bite'. As one writer has put it

> The English language is rich in the expression of how sexual and digestive pleasures are often related. Colloquial terms for a lover include: 'Honey', 'sweet', 'sugar'. The admission of sexual desire can take the words 'I could eat you up'. The practice of the love-bite probably stems from the unconscious urge to devour the partner.[57]

One might also see some aspects of oral sex within a similar context. Many writers have certainly noted the sexual implications of clinical vampiristic activity. The age-old link between vampirism and sex-

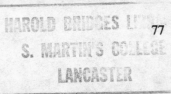

uality is well demonstrated in the legend surrounding the Rumanian vampire – Nosferatu – who is said to have combined his blood-sucking activities with rape.[58] Some of my respondents considered that vampiristic activity might well have its origins in, or be associated with, schizophrenic disorders of one kind or another. A number of them quoted instances in which paranoid patients had felt their blood was being drained from them (exsanguination) – a form of psychic vampirism. One or two also quoted cases in which such patients had indulged in auto-vampiristic activity. Occasionally, some severely mentally impaired patients have been reported as engaging in biting activities with accompanying blood ingestion. As already mentioned, biting, blood ingestion, and sometimes acts of serious mutilation may be the ingredients of sadistic sexual assaults committed by severely personality disordered individuals.[59]

Sometimes, such individuals have been reported as having indulged in blood drinking as part of 'black magic' and similar rituals. In my view this should not be regarded as vampirism in the more restricted clinical sense in which I am regarding it here. Whatever the causes, vampiristic activities seem to occur in persons functioning at a very 'primitive' mental and emotional level. It is, therefore, not altogether surprising that it is reported to be associated in some instances with schizoid, schizophrenic, or 'borderline' states. Those who espouse a psychoanalytic approach to such phenomena offer some interesting, if untestable, hypotheses. Thus, the phenomena have been likened to phantasies of biting, destruction, and possession of the mother of the tiny infant; indeed, Fenichel actually uses the word 'vampire' in this connection.[60] He suggests that such persons, who may be fixated at a very early stage of development, may well become those leech-like individuals who 'affix themselves ... [to others] ... by suction.'[61] Others have pointed to the central role of the teeth in vampiristic phenomena.

> The cutting of a child's teeth ... comes to assume a critical place in his emotional development, for if teeth can inflict pain on the mother, her teeth can also inflict pain on the child. When he later comes to expect retribution for his earlier cannibalistic tendencies, it is castration that is his unconscious fear.[62]

Some analysts have postulated that vampiristic and devouring behaviour may not only arise in response to severe maternal deprivation, but that it may also be seen in severe regression which some suggest is responsible for schizophrenic, schizoid, or borderline states. It has been held that the 'attack of the vampire' is consistent with some of the unconscious phantasies of schizophrenic persons ... (1) There is a partaking of life by the oral route using a sadistic attack by teeth, (2) the object is held and controlled while the vampire feeds, and finally (3) after feeding, the victim also becomes a vampire, indicating a merger between the feeder and the victim ... [63]

Metaphorically, and in the light of psychoanalytic theorising, the re-gressed schizophrenic, schizoid, or borderline personality has a tremendous need to be provided for and to be *nourished*. Perhaps he or she also has a compelling need to be provided with a form of mothering by those members of family and others who appear to have deprived them of such sustenance. The fear of exsanguination already referred to may well be an extension of these needs in their most severe form. The psychoanalytic view, incomplete and scientifi-cally untestable though it is, finds further support in the discussion of two cases by Vanden Bergh and Kelly and in more recent work on borderline personality disorders.[64] In the two cases in question (one of them an auto-vampirist), the patients had suffered from, or sub-sequently developed, a clear schizophrenic illness. The authors suggest that the ingestion of blood satisfied very basic oral-sadistic needs in their patients. They remark that the 'symbolic repre-sentation of the blood should always be investigated as an important clue to better understanding of the underlying pathology' (p. 547).

From a management point of view it is essential that attention be directed towards the main or underlying clinical condition so that this may be fully assessed and treated where possible. In those cases exhibiting gross personality disorder, and where this has resulted in homicidal activity or other serious violence against the person or persons, it will be necessary to secure the long-term detention of the individual in their own interests and those of society.

Summary and conclusion

On the basis of the available evidence from my small sample of re-spondents, and from an examination of the literature, it would appear that clinical vampirism is a fairly rare condition and that it is also highly likely to be associated with certain mental disorders such as the schizophrenias. However, there is also good reason for *suspect-ing* that the condition may not be quite as rare as some people suppose and that there are interesting if speculative links between the legendary and the clinical presentations. As one writer has suggested, 'that such dark images exist cannot be ignored, since beha-viour ... [emerges] ... which had hitherto been thought to exist only in folk-tale or myth ...'.[65] A Jungian conceptual framework might help us to link the two sets of phenomena more closely. For 'the world of the vampire has been described as a "twilight borderland where psychopathological and religious motives intermingle"'.[66]

Some other conditions and phenomena

The remainder of this chapter is devoted to certain other conditions and phenomena that seem to fit conveniently into the context of the preceding discussion; some may feel that their inclusion is a little arbitrary. The topics to be discussed are lycanthropy, zombiism, necrophilia, and certain aspects of serious sexual deviation.

Lycanthropy

> 'Even he who is pure of heart
> And says his prayers by night
> May become a wolf when the wolfbane blooms
> And the moon is full and bright.'
>
> (Ancient rhyme)

Linked with the legend of the vampire is that of the werewolf or, more correctly, the lycanthropic phenomenon. Strictly speaking, the term lycanthropy should only be appled to wolves or werewolves; however, it is also customarily applied to the condition in which a person believes he or she has been changed into an animal. The correct generic title is 'therianthropy'. The legend itself is age-old and ubiquitous. Its more positive aspect is seen in the ancient belief that the wolf was the protector of mankind; as such, it is exemplified in the Roman legend of Romulus and Remus, who were suckled by a wolf. The more malign elements of the legend possibly derive from the myths of the Norse gods who were said to take on animal forms such as those of bears or wolves. During the Middle Ages lycanthropic phenomena began to be associated with possession by evil spirits and the exercise of demonic powers. There is a legend that King John of England (1199–1216) was considered by some to have been a werewolf and that after his death the monks exhumed his body in order to give it sanctified rest.[67] In France, the phenomenon was known as *loupgarou*; legend has it that such a creature could be destroyed by taking drops of its blood during its 'wolf' period. One of the best known legendary methods of defeating the werewolf was to shoot it with bullets made of consecrated silver (such as those made from the silver crucifix from a church). It is of interest to compare this legend with that which probably lies behind the story of Weber's opera *Der Freischütz* (The Marksman) in which 'magic' bullets are used to defeat the powers of the Devil.

One of the earliest accounts of what appears to be a clinical presentation of lycanthropy is to be found in the Old Testament. Here, King Nebuchadnezzar is described as follows:

> He was banished from the society of men and ate grass like oxen; his body was drenched by the dew of heaven, until his hair grew long like goat's hair and his nails like eagle's talons.
>
> (*Daniel* 44: 33)

Chaucer also describes the troubled King's state very graphically in the Monk's Tale in *The Canterbury Tales*:

> And lyk a beste him seemed for to be,
> And eet hay as an oxe, and lay there-oute;
> ... and lyk an egle's featheres waxe his heres,
> His nayles lyk a briddes clawes were,
> Til God relessed him a certain yeres ...[68]

Both the biblical and Chaucer accounts indicate that his illness seems to have lasted several years and it is possible to infer that the disorder was associated with a depressive illness. The depressive element of lycanthropy had also been noted by Greek medical authorities such as Paulus Aegineta in the seventh century AD. For a long time, the condition seems to have been unresearched by psychiatric authorities. More recently, a revival of interest has taken place and a number of cases of lycanthropic phenomena have been reported in the clinical literature. In 1985 Coll *et al.* reviewed the literature during the previous ten years which revealed at least four cases. They then reported on a case of their own which concerned a woman of 66 who showed animal-like behaviour in which she would crawl and bark like a dog. She attributed her behaviour to the influence of demonic forces. She was treated by the use of drugs and ECT which resulted in a remission of her symptoms.[69]

In 1987, a report by the Medical Editor of the *Independent* newspaper described the case of a man who had been apprehended by the police having been brought to them by a frightened prostitute. She had complained that he had been acting strangely. He snarled at the police, crouched like a cornered animal, foamed at the mouth, and leaped at his pursuers. A senior police officer said 'The man was snarling, his lips were turned back and he held his hands rigid like claws. He seemed possessed of extraordinary strength and attacked the [policemen] with a ferocity that was frightening to all who observed him.' The man was taken to a psychiatric hospital and it was considered unlikely that he would be charged with any offence.[70] The author of the article, picking up on the possible sexual connotations found quite commonly in the clinical literature, puts forward such an explanation for the phenomenon. This is to the effect that lycanthropic behaviour often seems to have been precipitated by sexual intercourse. It is suggested, particularly by the psychoanalytically minded, that a person may become overwhelmed by chaotic fears and sexual feelings which are then expressed in this bizarre animalistic fashion. Jung once described a case of lycanthropy in which two daughters consistently dreamed of their mother being transformed into an animal. He suggested that when, many years later, the mother actually developed lycanthropic symptoms during a psychotic illness, this reflected the emergence of primitive drives, long repressed, which were recognised earlier in the unconscious of her daughters through their dreams. (Compare this with my earlier comments on a Jungian approach to the phenomenon of the vampire.)[71] In 1988 Fahy *et al.* outlined several cases in which lycanthropic presentations were features of depressive and schizophreniform illnesses. In two of the cases there were sexual components similar to those suggested above.[72]

In 1988 Keck *et al.* sought to demonstrate that lycanthropy was 'alive and well in the twentieth century'.[73] They conducted a review of some 5,000 cases that had been admitted to a private 250-bedded psychiatric facility in Boston, Massachusetts during a 12-year period. They found 12 cases in which the features of lycanthropy had persisted for periods ranging from 1 day to 13 years. The patients' ages ranged from 16–38; ten were male and two female. They selected the following operational definition to include at least one of the following. That: '(1) The individual reported verbally, during intervals of lucidity or retrospectively, that he or she was a particular animal. (2) The individual behaved in a manner reminiscent of a particular animal; i.e. howling, growling, crawling on all fours.' The researchers examined four of the patients during their actual episodes and interviewed three others retrospectively. In the remaining five cases, one or more members of the nursing staff who had witnessed the behaviour were interviewed. The animals represented in the group included wolf, gerbil, dog, cat, bird, rabbit, and tiger. All twelve of the patients were treated with drugs. Seven appeared to have experienced full remission of symptoms, three partial remission and one remained unchanged. The latter case had been in various treatments for his condition for over six years. Nine cases were diagnosed as suffering from bipolar affective disorder, two from schizophrenia, and one from a borderline personality disorder. This quite recent study seems to be one of the most comprehensive to have appeared. As the authors suggest, the condition appears to occur in a setting of major psychiatric disorder yet the delusions have a monosymptomatic quality about them (see also Chapter three). Some authorities have suggested that because, in recent times, the existence of wolves in Europe seems to have decreased, cases of lycanthropy may have become virtually non-existent. As the authors suggest, 'lycanthropy persists as an occasional but colourful feature of severe, and occasionally factitious, psychosis. However, it appears that the delusion of being transformed into an animal may bode no more ill than any other delusion' (p. 119).

Zombiism

> '... and the dead shall be rais'd ... and we shall be chang'd.'
> (1 *Corinthians* 15: 52–53)

In some parts of the world, but most notably in Haiti, there is a very powerful belief that a priest/magician (bocor/bokor/Houngan) can restore the dead to life and have them used as slaves (Zombies). Strictly speaking a bokor appears to be one who practises sorcery as a profession and a Houngan is a Voudoun priest. It appears the titles are often used synonymously. It is important to stress that this belief has its roots in a country that is beset by much poverty and internal strife. As I noted in the discussion of possession states in Chapter four and in the discussion of vampirism above, such conditions are fertile soil for the generation of such folk beliefs, where it is often difficult to draw a firm dividing line between myth and reality. It is also important to stress that the word Zombi, which in popular belief represents a reanimated corpse, has a variety of other meanings.[74] For many years it had been believed that there might well be a physical explanation for this so-called supernatural phenomenon.[75] Recent work has suggested that the ingestion of a variety of powerful poisons, administered with considerable skill, could account for the phenomenon. A young ethno-biologist, Wade Davis, with a good grounding in modern pharmacology and toxicology, carried out a lengthy field investigation into the matter. Although some of his work has been criticised, it would seem that his findings may help to provide an explanation. The simplified essence of his findings is as follows. Victims are administered poison derived from one or more species of the puffer fish which contains the constituent tetrodotoxin.[76] (Poisons from certain other sources were also identified, for example, a local toad.) This results in a state of complete paralysis (catalepsy), yet, at the same time, a full awareness of what is happening. It would thus be very easy for the person to be declared dead. Following speedy exhumation and resuscitation, the victim is then given the powerful hallucinogenic compound, datura. This is said to account for the trance-like state that is seen in the victims, for their loss of memory of what has happened, and for their willingness to work subsequently as 'slaves'. Wade Davis has not only published an extensive account of his researches for a popular readership, but has also presented his findings in the relevant learned journals.[77] Though not without its critics, his work indicates that continuing serious study should be given to confirming a scientific explanation for the 'living dead' of peasant folk-lore. Should his findings receive further confirmation, they have important implications for further research into the physical explanations that have been offered in the past for vampirism and allied phenomena.

Necrophilia

> '... Defaced, deflowered, and now to death devote!'
> (Milton, *Paradise Lost*, Book 9)

The term 'necrophilia' (from the Greek *nekros* (corpse) and *philia* (love)) has been given a variety of meanings. It is generally taken to mean molestation of, or sexual relations with, cadavers and in a wider sense has also been used to mean a morbid interest in death and in funeral rites.[78] When using the term, most people mean *sexual* as distinct from *non-sexual* necrophilia, which should be confined to handling, gazing upon, or dismembering corpses. However, it is often difficult to draw hard and fast boundaries between the various activities.[79] Mythology and folk-lore contain many references to necrophilic behaviour. Achilles is said to have violated the corpse of an Amazon queen and Periander is said to have sexually abused the body of his dead wife. There are also necrophilic themes in some nursery tales – such as *Sleeping Beauty*. Literature also has its examples of necrophilia; for example, in *Romeo and Juliet* and in *Wuthering Heights*. History, both ancient and more recent, affords examples of necrophilic behaviour. In ancient Egypt, it is said that certain male embalmers forsook their professional standards and were caught sexually molesting the corpses of attractive high-born women. Not only were the offenders punished, but the embalming of such females was handed over to female embalmers. In addition, embalming was delayed for several days, presumably in the hope that putrefaction would render such activities less attractive! In the Middle Ages, it was the practice, in some places, for monks to keep vigil over the corpses of the nobility. Some monks were said to have abused their trust and violated female corpses. It may be that the Orthodox Jewish custom of having a 'watcher' over the dead body – to keep vigil – has similar origins.

In Central Europe until some 200 years ago it was said that if a betrothed girl died before her nuptial day could be celebrated, the bridegroom could still consummate the rite by having sexual relations with the body. In some parts of the world, in less developed communities, sexual congress with corpses is said to be practised as part of certain initiation and magical ceremonies. It is also of interest to note that corpses have often been invested with special healing powers; for example, the ancient practice of pressing a corpse's finger on an aching tooth. Pliny recorded the efficacy of a corpse's hand as follows:

> Stroking with the hand of a person who has died early is supposed to cure goitre, glandular swellings near the ear, and throat complaints; nevertheless, a good many think that this can be effected by any corpse's hand, provided only that the dead person be of the same sex and the thing is done with the left hand up-turned.[80]

Some case illustrations

Some sadistic murderers are alleged to have indulged in necrophilic activity, thus confirming how difficult it is to place behaviour into neat and discrete categories. Examples are the infamous killer of children, the Count Gilles de Rais, Gamier, Leger, Sergeant Bertrand, Peter Kurten, Fritz Haarman, and Albert Fish. In the U.K. Christie, the notorious Rillington Place murderer, appears to have carried out necrophilic activities on some of the women he murdered. The evidence from pathologists showed that sexual intercourse had taken place at or shortly after death.[81] In America, a notorious case was that of Kemper, described by Smith and Dimock.[82] Kemper had been incarcerated in a mental hospital for killing his grandparents. He was released and later admitted to several killings. He would take off the dead female victim's clothes, gaze upon the body, sometimes photograph it, and then have sex. Sometimes he would also commit sexual acts with parts of the corpses after dismemberment. He eventually gave himself up to the authorities and was subsequently sentenced to life imprisonment. More recently, the case of Dennis Nilsen has aroused interest in this country. Nilsen admitted to killing fifteen young men and then dissecting, boiling, and burning some of their bodies as a means of disposal. A plea of diminished responsibility on the grounds of an abnormality of mind failed, and he was sentenced to life imprisonment with a recommendation from the judge that he serve a minimum of twenty-five years.

Nilsen sometimes sought his companions for sexual purposes, sometimes merely for their company. For present purposes, what is more relevant is that the evidence in his case suggests that he sometimes committed necrophilic acts, like undressing the corpse, laying it out to his liking, and then gazing upon it. Of even more interest is the fact that he would take steps to make himself look like a corpse by powdering himself to imitate the pallor of death. Having done this, he would lie down beside the corpse of his victim. It would appear that Nilsen could only find real sexual solace in the company of an inanimate partner.[83] Sometimes, the necrophilic tendencies lead the offender to take more violent steps in order to seek satisfaction. In a case reported upon in 1985, a man received a sentence of four years' imprisonment for mutilating corpses. (It is of interest to note that there is no statute that covers necrophilia as a specific sexual offence.) When his house was searched police found a photograph of a man's severed genitalia. He admitted mutilating three bodies and allegedly told the police that, for a long time, he had nursed a phantasy of cutting off male genitalia.[84] In some cases, it is difficult to determine whether a murder has been committed solely for the purpose of sexual molestation after death. One example is a case in which the offender lived out his necrophilic phantasies by first killing and then sexually molesting his young male victim. He then disposed of the body down a mine-shaft.[85] The authors of this case report also describe a further case in which it was strongly suspected, but not proved, that necrophilic activity had been committed after the murder of a 9-year-old boy. In another case a man indicted for murder confessed, in the course of police enquiries, to breaking into a mortuary and attempting sexual relations with female corpses.[86]

Explanations

Persons who commit necrophilic acts will have grossly disordered personalities. Some may be suffering from psychotic states, such as schizophrenia, and others may be of impaired intelligence. However, in the case of the man who confessed during police enquiries to sexual molestation of female corpses, he is reputed to have had a very high I.Q. In a number of case reports serious alcohol abuse has been implicated. Indeed, in the case of Nilsen, a psychiatrist writing a postscript to Brian Masters' book suggested that the latter had probably under-estimated the important part played by alcohol in disinhibiting Nilsen, thus enabling him to live with the grisly products of his bizarre activities.[87] Psychoanalysts have not been slow to proffer explanations for understanding this very bizarre form of human behaviour. It has been suggested that it is due to a need to bring about a reunion with a mother-figure linked with the involvement of sadistic elements. The sexual role played by an entirely helpless victim, and the parts played by a primitive form of curiosity and exploration, are also important. Other such explanations have included attempts to compensate for castration anxiety, the need to overcome physical inadequacy, and a fear of relationships with women. There are obvious connections between other seriously sexually deviant activities such as sexual murder, bondage-type behaviours, and sexually induced asphyxia, some aspects of which I shall now consider.

Sexual murder and other matters

'I will kill thee and love thee after.'
(*Othello*, Act V, Scene ii)

It is difficult to estimate the annual number of murders that are clearly sexually motivated since the term 'sexual murder' covers a very wide range of behaviours. It is also possible that some murders may be sexually motivated but that this is not apparent on first inspection. For the purpose of this brief discussion I am not including *crimes passionnels* (hetero- and homosexual) but only those cases where some form of serious sexual deviation and aggression is associated with the killing. It has been calculated that in 1984 some 8 per cent of homicides could be classified in this way.[88] An earlier study quoted by the same author indicates that of 306 murders of females over 16 years of age, 14 per cent were thought to be sexually motivated. Sexual murders, particularly of children (of which there are fortunately still only a very small number), arouse strong feelings amongst those concerned with the detection of the culprits and the general public. In cases of sexual murder (and others) the police sometimes seek the help of psychologists and psychiatrists in trying to build a psychological 'profile' of the killer. This profiling has become popular in the United States.[89] It includes practical matters such as details about the death(s), location of the body, and evidence of attempted or actual intercourse. It also includes such questions as, do the wounds suggest the infliction of torture as part of the assault as an aid to sexual pleasure? If there has been mutilation of the body, has this also been part of the sexual behaviour, or carried out as a means of preventing identification of the victim? Such profiling would then go on to try to determine psychological motives such as lust, desire to shock, or to get even with society. If such characteristics are present it is likely that the assailant may be known locally as a troublemaker and perhaps be at odds with both family and the community. It has been suggested also that such a person might appear to be careful and cunning in the commission of his crime, but that he might also give himself away by showing undue interest in the case or, like some arsonists, by volunteering help and/or information.[90]

As already suggested, sexual murder is a fairly rare event and the motivation behind it is often unclear. Did the murder occur as a result of the pursuit of sadistic sexual pleasure or as a means of rendering the victim unable to give evidence? Was it the result of an unintentional act of violence that had become lethal during some form of sexual activity? For example, it is possible for manual strangulation to occur during some forms of anal intercourse; it is also possible for death to occur in the course of fellatio due to aspiration of ejaculate or from impaction of the penis in the hypopharynx. Certain groups of individuals may be especially vulnerable to serious sexual attack, notably children and the elderly because of their physical vulnerability, female and male prostitutes, and promiscuous persons of both sexes.

Motivation

As indicated, the motivation for sexual murder may be very complex. One authority has stressed the manner in which different facets of the sexual murderer's personality may seem to be out of touch with one another. Kindness and compassion can co-exist with a high degree of cruelty and savage destructiveness. Such persons would appear to have a capacity to 'split off' feelings from behaviour; such a capacity is seen in the seriously psychopathic and in some hysterical personalities. Such highly pathological behaviour is graphically described by Cox in his reference to the sadistic sexual murder of the King in Marlowe's play *Edward II*. The illustration concerns the use of the red-hot spit that is used to penetrate the King anally and which results in his agonising and lingering death. The red-hot spit is used in combination with a table to stamp on him, 'But not too hard, lest that you bruise his body'.[91] At a superficial level it may be that such activity was carried out to avoid easy visual identification of the King's injuries, but at a deeper level, it would seem highly suggestive of the jarring incompatibilities of behaviour suggested earlier. Few experts have provided adequate 'pen portraits' of the sadistic sexual murderer. One exception was the late Dr Robert Brittain who had the combined professional expertise and experience of the forensic pathologist and psychiatrist.[92] It is important to emphasise that Brittain only suggested a *composite* picture; we should not expect to find all the many features he described in any one case. The following is a selection of some of the characteristics. Such persons are often withdrawn, introverted, over-controlled, and even quite timid. Some, strangely enough, are even prudish and may take offence at the telling of 'dirty jokes'. Such killers are likely to be about 30 or older and they may come from a variety of occupations. A surprising number have worked in the butchery trade or been employed in abattoirs. Nilsen, referred to earlier, may have learned his dismemberment skills in his work as a 'cook and butcher' in the army. Sexual murderers often seem to be remarkably ambivalent towards their mothers – the devoted son on the one hand and the mother-hater on the other. This is a view expressed by many psychoanalytically orientated authorities. In other words, their personalities show a mass of contradictions with many unresolved psychological conflicts. The mothers of such killers tend to be gentle and over-indulgent, whilst the fathers are often found to be rigidly strict or absent. Such offenders often have an active and bizarre phantasy life; such phantasies are sometimes used as a means of rehearsal for a future killing. Their phantasies are often enhanced by a preoccupation with violent and sadistic pornography and they are likely to show a marked interest in torture and atrocities, Nazi activities, horror films, black magic, and the occult. They also tend to be unreasonably preoccupied with the size of their genitalia and their sex lives are often poor or non-existent. The murder may be planned over several weeks or months and, as already indicated, such offenders seem quite lacking in remorse for the appalling injuries they inflict.[93] In some cases, the sight of their helpless victims may well serve to heighten their sexual arousal and lead them to repeated frenzied attacks. Asphyxia is a common method of sadistic sexual killing, since by this means the victim's suffering may be prolonged. They may be rendered unconscious by strangulation, brought round, rendered unconscious again and so on. The victim is therefore quite powerless – as though in the power of a malevolent spider. Contrary to popular belief, sexual intercourse or, for that matter, any sexual activity with the victim, may not necessarily accompany the murder. It has been suggested that such murders may be a *substitute* for sexual activity.[94] However, these offenders may masturbate by the side of the body or merely gaze at it. The practices that accompany the killing or that actually cause the death are often horrendous. The offender may insert an object such as a torch, milk bottle, or poker with great force into the victim's vagina or rectum. A good illustration of such behaviour was that shown by Neville Heath who was hanged for the sadistic sexual killing of two women. He had inserted objects into their vaginas with tremendous force. The prognosis for such offenders is not good. Those in charge of them and who share the responsibility for making recommendations about future dangerousness have to guard against being misled by *appearances* of good behaviour and apparently sincere protestations of reform. Many such offenders have a tendency to repeat their acts of sexual aggression – even after many years of institutionalisation. On the other hand, some of them have an awareness of the powerful nature of their deviant desires and drives. They are sometimes frightened of their sadistic impulses and activities and are grateful for the containment offered them by a secure hospital or penal establishment.[95]

Ritual murder

One should also note briefly the phenomenon of ritual murder in which there is often a major sexual element. Ritual murders may involve the mutilation or removal of sex organs such as the penis, testicles, vagina, or the breasts. Cases have been reported in southern Nigeria and in Ghana. One outbreak occurred in which men disguised themselves as leopards to make the killings look like the activity of animals. This was possible in a setting in which there was an active belief in lycanthropic phenomena. Some of the causes attributed to such ritual killings in Nigeria can be summarised as follows: (1) as a request for divine assistance in warfare; (2) a search for rain and a good harvest; (3) as a sacrifice to secure peace; (4) to increase individual wealth; (5) as a means of averting disasters or epidemics; (6) to placate the gods; (7) to establish or reinforce a community taboo.

Such killings are yet another example of the need to see 'clinical' phenomena against a background of culture, myth, and folk-lore.[96]

Sexuality and fatality

> 'Let's hang ourselves immediately!'
> (Samuel Beckett, *Waiting for Godot*)

Reference has already been made to the manner in which death may occur by 'accident' during sexual activity. Such activity does not have to be deviant for death to occur. Any activity involving strenuous physical exertion like sex brings attendant risks. However, I now wish to consider some behaviours that, by their very nature, provide more than a slight risk of fatality; indeed, one element in the practices to be described could be said to represent 'dicing with death'. Sexual excitement and orgasm can, of course, be produced in a variety of ways. One of the stranger methods is that of self-induced asphyxiation (eroticised repetitive hanging). Bizarre though such behaviour may seem, it is not apparently so rare as may be imagined. Figures for the United States suggest some 50 cases per year. There do not appear to be comparable figures for the U.K. but, as I shall show shortly, cases are occasionally reported in the medical and forensic literature. The production of erection and orgasm by hanging are to be found in the world's great literature. There are accounts by de Sade (*Justine*), and the quotation used at the heading of this section is taken from a longer extract from *Waiting for Godot*, where hanging and ejaculation are discussed by the characters Estragon and Vladimir. A contemporary of J.S. Bach, the musician Kotzwarra (whose name is sometimes used to describe the condition – Kotzwarra syndrome), died as a result of such activity. He had persuaded a prostitute to suspend him. Unfortunately, the suspension exceeded the time that Kotzwarra anticipated would bring about the required sexual satisfaction and he died. The prostitute was tried for murder, but fortunately acquitted. Reports of such activity have been reported world-wide, amongst some Eskimo populations and in various parts of South America. The methods used to bring about such sexual pleasure are many and varied. They consist mainly of the use of various hanging contrivances, some of which are very esoteric. Sometimes drugs are used to heighten the experience; for example, amyl nitrite ('poppers') which heightens orgasm. The physiological processes involved in producing such states of sexual excitement and arousal are highly complex and well described in the literature.[97] An associated sado-masochistic phenomenon is that of *bondage*. Here the 'victim' either ties himself up or is tied up in very complicated ways by a variety of methods. Ropes, straps, and chains all have their vogues. There are magazines specially devoted to such activity and, in the United States, there is an 'underground' where like-minded indulgers may get in touch with one another. It has been estimated that in the U.S.A. some 250 deaths occur by this means each year. Once in the bondage state, the 'victim' may also induce his partner or partners to subject him to various forms of humiliation; examples are: being urinated on or excreted over, whipped, or otherwise chastised. Nearly all such sado-masochistic individuals are male, though there are a few very rare reports of females being involved. Females are much more likely to be used as aggressors; indeed some prostitutes are said to specialise in this kind of activity. Many sado-masochists are lonely, isolated men and are often depressed. There appears to be no typical family pathology, but often poor family relationships are evident. One explanation proffered is that the person needs to be punished for some early unresolved infantile guilt. Castration anxiety has also been offered as an explanation in some cases. For others, it would seem that the 'risk' element is highly attractive and the bizarre nature of the activity probably adds a heightened excitement to lives that are sometimes drab or unhappy. Others have seen the behaviour as a suicidal syndrome; 'it would seem appropriate to consider this as a suicidal syndrome of life threatening behaviour, involving erotisation of dying brought about in order to escape overwhelming anxiety, rather than "accidental death".'[98] One or two cases from the U.K. literature emphasise the difficulty in deciding whether deaths from such activity are in fact suicidal or accidental. In one case, a man of 25 was found hanging from a tree in a wood. The circumstances surrounding the case suggested that, although this was clearly a masochistic act (the body was naked and the position of the ropes was typical of bondage practice), there were also strong indications of suicidal intention, though the Coroner's verdict was of 'accidental death'.[99] The author describes three further cases in which, although masochistic practices were apparent, there was 'probably or inevitably an expectation of death occurring'. The writer also makes the important point that true asphyxia is by no means always present, 'death frequently occurring from reflex cardiac arrest owing to pressure on the neck ...'. Sometimes other means for obtaining sexual pleasure are used – with fatal consequences. Sivaloganathan suggests that, although the commonest activity appears to be asphyxial death, with or without the application of plastic bags or the inhalation of volatile liquids (which may be used to enhance the erotic effect), there are other methods. He describes a case in which a young man was found dead with a wire cradle attached to his scrotum and another wire inserted in his anus. The wires had been connected to a low electricity source (the loudspeaker in the T.V. set). His death occurred when he went to see why no current was coming through his contrived source of sexual stimulation. In doing so, the side of his face had come into contact with a live part of the T.V. set containing very high voltage. It was *this* that had resulted in his death.[100] In a later paper this author describes an unusual case of auto-erotic drowning. A man of 36 was discovered dead at the bottom of a river. He was tied in typical auto-erotic fashion. His clothing also indicated transvestite interests. The scene of the fatality and other evidence suggested that

the deceased [had] used a novel method of producing asphyxia ... by submerging himself in the water and achieving stimulation by partial drowning ... it would appear that he would tie himself *relatively loosely* [my italics] with ligatures and tie his feet to a heavy stone with the aid of a clothes-line and then submerge himself, armed with a pair of scissors.

When he thought he had had enough stimulation, he would use the scissors to cut himself free. On the last occasion he had been unable to release himself – with fatal results.[101] More recently, Ikeda *et al.* have reported upon a case from Japan. In this instance a man, aged 25, used a number of articles of clothing (three skirts, a pinafore dress, a pair of panty hose and a plastic bag) to induce auto-erotic suffocation; sadly this ended in his death.[102]

Concluding comment

A variety of deviant and unusual practices have been surveyed briefly in this chapter. Inevitably I have had to be selective and there are a number of omissions. I have not considered zoophilia (sexual relations with animals); coprophilia and related phenomena (sexual arousal produced by excrement or defecation; urination (urolagnia); or sexual excitement caused by having an enema (klismaphilia). Those who wish to pursue these and other rare disorders will find useful sources in the extensive literature I have quoted.

Notes and references

Some of the material contained in this chapter appeared in my paper 'Vampirism – Legendary or Clinical Phenomenon?', *Medicine, Science and the Law*, 1984, vol. 24, pp. 283–293. It is reproduced here by kind permission of the editor and the publishers.

1. R.E. Hemphill and T. Zabow, 'Clinical Vampirism: A Presentation of 3 Cases and a Re-evaluation of Haigh, the "Acid-bath Murderer"', *South African Medical Journal*, 1983, vol. 63, pp. 278–281. A very short account of this research was published in *The Times*, 6 May 1983.
2. H. Prins, *The Times*, 19 May 1983.
3. W.L. Neustatter, *The Mind of the Murderer*, London, Christopher Johnson, 1957, Chapter 11. It would appear that Haigh *himself* did not seek an insanity defence. Hemphill, personal communication, 10 November 1984.
4. A much shorter account for a more general psychiatric readership appeared in the *British Journal of Psychiatry*. See H. Prins, 'Vampirism – A Clinical Condition', *British Journal of Psychiatry*, 1985, vol. 146, pp. 666–668.

5. For a fascinating account of the history of aphrodisiacs see P.V. Taberner, *Aphrodisiacs: The Science and the Myth*, London, Croom Helm, 1985.

6. For an account of some such uses, and other more esoteric medicinal practices see B. Walker, *Encyclopaedia of Metaphysical Medicine*, London, Routledge and Kegan Paul, 1978.

7. Walker, op. cit. 1978, p. 253.

8. Walker, op. cit. See also A. Masters, *Natural History of the Vampire*, London, Rupert and Hart Davis, 1972.

9. P. Barker, 'On the Melodrama, and Tragedy of Aids', *Independent Magazine*, 26 November 1988. p. 14. Similar suppositions can be made about attitudes towards venereal disease. See, for example, J.S. Cummings, 'Pox and Paranoia in Renaissance Europe', *History Today*, 1989, January, pp. 28–35. Addressing a similar theme, I suggested in a letter to the *Independent* of 30 December 1986 that we could not address subjects such as AIDS unless we 'were mindful of the context in which fear surrounding such an illness can give rise to such emotive expressions as "war on AIDS", "cesspits" and the like'. I also made the point that knowledge derived from history and anthropology 'reveals that fear and mystery have always been associated with the secretion and dissemination of bodily fluids – particularly blood and semen. These fears have given rise to powerful myths (the ubiquitous, ancient, but long-standing myth of the vampire is but one example).'

10. R. Titmuss, *The Gift Relationship: From Human Blood to Social Policy*, London, Allen and Unwin, 1970, p. 15.

11. Titmuss, op. cit. 1970, p. 15.

12. See D.O. Topp, 'Fire as a Symbol and as a Weapon of Death', *Medicine, Science and the Law*, 1973, vol. 13, pp. 79–86.

13. See M. Summers, *The Vampire in Europe*, Wellingborough, Aquarian Press, 1980.

14. Reported in the *Independent*, 6 October 1987. The existence of large amounts of blood was revealed by 'chemical tests on a six foot deep band of black earth at the site of a monastic hospital at Soutra, Lothian'.

15. See, for example, C. Lévi-Strauss, *Structural Anthropology*, Harmondsworth, Penguin Books, 1972. The topic is also addressed by Mary Douglas. See in particular, M. Douglas, *Purity and Danger: An Analysis of the Concepts of Pollution and Taboo*, London, Ark Paperbacks, 1984. Also M. Douglas, *Natural Symbols: Explorations in Cosmology*, Harmondsworth, Penguin Education, 1978.

16. J.G. Frazer, *The Golden Bough* (abridged edition), London, Macmillan, 1949. See also B.G. Burton-Bradley, 'Cannibalism for Cargo', *Journal of Nervous and Mental Diseases*, 1976, vol. 163, pp. 428–431.

17. J. Shinner, 'For Happiness and Fertility, Feast an Ancestor', *Independent*, 9 August 1988. Recent archaeological investigation of U.K. Stone Age burials suggests that cannibalism was probably practised though the evidence is not conclusive. The *Independent*, 15

April 1987 and 28 July 1987. Cannibalism is also discussed usefully in T. Fahy, S. Wesseley and A. David, 'Werewolves, Vampires and Cannibals', *Medicine, Science and the Law*, 1988, vol. 28, pp. 145–149.

18. A.R. Favazza, *Bodies Under Siege: Self-Mutilation in Culture and Society*, London, Johns Hopkins University Press, 1987, p. 6.
19. P. Loizes, personal communication, 1983.
20. M. Benezech, M. Bourgeois, D. Boukhabza and J. Yesavage, 'Cannibalism and Vampirism in Paranoid Schizophrenia', *Journal of Clinical Psychiatry*, 1981, vol. 42, p. 290.
21. M. Benezech *et al.*, op. cit. 1981, p. 290.
22. See R. Favazza, op. cit. 1987, pp. 95–99. The author also provides examples of a variety of practices from a number of other cultures.
23. I am grateful to Mr. R.S. Levy for comment on this topic. Personal communication, February 1985. For an illustration of the taboo of menstrually soiled cloths in developing countries see J. Stevens, 'Brief Psychoses: Do They Contribute to the Good Prognosis and Equal Prevalence of Schizophrenia in Developing Countries?', *British Journal of Psychiatry*, 1987, vol. 151, pp. 393–396.
24. For further discussion see L. Kayton, 'The Relationship of the Vampire Legend to Schizophrenia', *Journal of Youth and Adolescence*, 1972, vol. 1, pp. 303–314. R.H. Robbins, The Encyclopaedia of Witchcraft and Demonology, Feltham, Newnes Books, 1984, pp. 521–525. L. Spence, *An Encyclopaedia of Occultism*, London, Routledge, Kegan Paul, Trench and Trubner, 1920. A. Calmet, *Dissertation sur Les Apparitions des Esprits et sur Les Vampires et Revenants*, 1749. Extracted and translated in Chapter I of O. Volta and V. Riva, *The Vampire: An Anthology*, London, Pan Books, 1965.
25. J. Du Bulay, 'The Greek Vampire: A Study of Cyclic Symbolism in Marriage and Death', *Man: Journal of the Royal Anthropological Institute* (New Series), 1982, vol. 17, pp. 219–238.
26. See Spence, op. cit. 1920.
27. See M. Summers, *The Vampire: His Kith and Kin*, New York, University Books, 1960; M. Summers, *The Vampire in Europe*, Wellingborough, Aquarian Press, 1980; M. Summers, *The History of Witchcraft and Demonology*, London, Routledge and Kegan Paul, 1973.
28. M. Summers, *The Vampire in Europe*, pp. xx–xxi.
29. M. Summers, *The Galanty Show: An Autobiography by Montague Summers*, London, Cecil Woolf, 1980.
30. Michael Cox in Foreword to Summers, *The Vampire in Europe*, op. cit. 1980, p. xvii.
31. M. Summers, *The Vampire in Europe*, op. cit., p. 288.
32. Rev. R. Grainger, personal communication, July 1983.
33. P. Barber, *Vampires, Burial and Death: Folklore and Reality*, London, Yale University Press, 1988.
34. C. Leatherdale, *Dracula: The Novel and the Legend, A Study of Bram Stoker's Gothic Masterpiece*, Wellingborough, Aquarian Press, 1985. The power of novels and films to fuel the myth and the need for it has

been recently described briefly by Pullinger. See K. Pullinger, 'My Hero, Kate Pullinger on Dracula', *Independent Magazine*, 24 June 1989.

35. A. Ryan (ed.), *The Penguin Book of Vampire Stories*, Harmondsworth, Penguin Books, 1988.

36. From P. Barber, op. cit., p. 88. Reproduced by kind permission of the publishers, Yale University Press.

37. A psychiatrist colleague of mine, who has a particular interest in this topic, has pointed out in a letter to the *British Journal of Psychiatry* that the particular variant of porphyria, if it had any importance at all, was probably the recessively inherited congenital condition, found not infrequently in South Africa. It was not likely to have been the variant of the disease known as *erythropoietic protoporphyria* that I had assumed to be the case in my own study of the topic (Prins, op. cit. 1984). My colleague also makes the important point that if certain disorders are sensationalised this may be harmful to genuine sufferers from such conditions, a point with which I agree entirely. See K. De Pauw, Letter, *British Journal of Psychiatry*, 1984, vol. 147, p. 320. See also R.S. Day, 'Bloodlust, Madness, and the Press', *New Scientist*, 1984, 13 September pp. 53–54.

38. The most persuasive recent exponent of the porphyria connection appears to be Professor David Dolphin in an unpublished lecture entitled 'Werewolves and Vampires' given to a meeting of the American Association for the Advancement of Science in 1985. I am grateful to Professor Dolphin for providing me with an abstract of his address (25.6.85). For a general account of porphyria see G. Dean, *The Porphyrias – A Story of Inheritance and Environment* (2nd edn), London, Pitman, 1971, and L. Illis, 'On Porphyria and the Aetiology of Werewolves', *Proceedings of the Royal Society of Medicine*, 1964, vol. 57, pp. 23–26. For more recent comment on work in this area see L. Milgrom, 'Vampires, Plants and Crazy Kings', *New Scientist*, 26 April 1984, pp. 9–13. Barber, op. cit. 1988, pp. 99–100 reviews some of the recent work and tends to dismiss its relevance. The use of garlic was given an interesting contemporary twist recently. Anthony Sher, in his portrayal of Malvolio (Royal Shakespeare Company, Stratford, 11 February 1987), has him use a cross *and garlic* in attempting to deal with his so-called 'madness'.

39. Dr J.M. Dunlop, personal communication, 1987. I am grateful to Dr Dunlop for many helpful observations on the topics of vampirism and associated conditions.

40. For an extension of these views see, for example, E. Jones, *On the Nightmare*, New York, Liveright, 1951.

41. See D. Farson and A. Hall, *Mysterious Monsters* (enlarged edn), London, Aldous Books, 1978. The point is also developed by J.M. Dunlop. See J.M. Dunlop, 'Genetic Engineering – A Waste of Valuable Resources?', *Public Health*, London 1974, vol. 89, pp. 13–17.

42. See Spence, op. cit. 1920, and Robbins, op. cit. 1984, for some

illustrations.

43. Dr J. Coid, personal communication, 12.8.86.
44. *Independent*, 14 April 1987.
45. *Daily Mail*, 26 October 1985 and *Daily Express*, 25 October 1985.
46. *Guardian*, 12 December 1987.
47. *Independent*, 3 December 1987.
48. *Sunday Sport*, 12 June 1988.
49. *Independent*, 1 June 1989.
50. Hemphill and Zabow, op. cit. 1983, p. 278.
51. See in particular E.F. Sharpe, *Collected Papers on Psychoanalysis*, London, Hogarth Press, 1950 (notably Chapter IV), and G. Fellion, J.P. Duflot, P.Anglade and J. Fraillon, 'From Fantasy to Reality: On Criminal and Cannibalistic Behaviour', *Annales Medico-Psychologiques*, 1980, vol. 138, pp. 596–602.
52. A. Bourguignon, 'Vampirism and Auto-Vampirism', in L.B. Schlesinger and E. Revitch (eds), *Sexual Dynamics of Anti-Social Behaviour*, Springfield, Illinois, Charles C. Thomas, 1983, pp. 278–301.
53. See Walker, op. cit. 1978, and Burton-Bradley, op. cit. 1976.
54. See, for example, R.L. Vanden Bergh and J.F. Kelly, 'Vampirism – A Review With New Observations', *Archives of General Psychiatry*, 1964, vol. 11, pp. 543–547, and R. Von Krafft-Ebing, *Psychopathia Sexualis*, New York, Scarborough Books, 1978.
55. A. Bartholomew, 'Two Features Associated With Intravenous Drug Users: A Note', *Australian and New Zealand Journal of Psychiatry*, 1973, vol. 7, pp. 1–2.
56. J.S. Kwawer, 'Some Interpersonal Aspects of Self-mutilation in a Borderline Patient', *Journal of the American Academy of Psychoanalysis*, 1980, vol. 8, pp. 203–216. On self-mutilation more generally see A.R. Favazza, op. cit.
57. See Leatherdale, op. cit. 1986, p. 161. The use of oral sexual practices between males in order to gain virility and as a means of maintaining social reciprocity is evidenced in the phallocentric activities of some dwellers in New Guinea. See T. Schneebaum, *Where the Spirits Dwell*, London, Weidenfeld and Nicolson, 1988.
58. See Bourguignon, op. cit. 1983.
59. See R.P. Brittain, 'The Sadistic Murderer', *Medicine, Science and the Law*, 1970, vol. 10, pp. 198–207.
60. O. Fenichel, *The Psychoanalytic Theory of Neurosis*, London, Routledge and Kegan Paul, 1978, p. 65.
61. Fenichel, op. cit. 1978, p. 489.
62. Leatherdale, op. cit. 1986, p. 166.
63. Kayton, op. cit. 1972, p. 310.
64. Vanden Bergh and Kelly, op. cit. 1964, p. 547. For a survey of more recent work on borderline states see P.L.G. Gallway, 'The Psycho-dynamics of Borderline Personality', in D.P. Farrington and J. Gunn (eds), *Aggression and Dangerousness*, Chichester, John Wiley, 1985.
65. R.S. McCully, 'Vampirism: Historical Perspective and Underlying

Process in Relation to a Case of Auto-vampirism', *Journal of Nervous and Mental Diseases*, 1964, vol. 139, pp. 440–452. p. 447. See more recently A. Halevy, Y. Levi, A. Shnaker and R. Orda, 'Auto-vampirism – An Unusual Case of Anaemia', *Journal of the Royal Society of Medicine*, 1989, vol. 82, pp. 630–631.

66. G. Nandris, 'The Historical Dracula: The Theme of His Legend in the Western and in the Eastern Literatures of Europe', *Comparative Literature Studies*, 1966, vol. 3, pp. 392–393 (quoted in Leatherdale, op. cit. 1986, at p. 175).

67. Reader's Digest Association, *Reader's Digest of Strange Stories, Amazing Facts*, London, 1976.

68. G. Chaucer, *Complete Works* (edited by W.W. Skeat), London, Oxford University Press, 1951. p. 534.

69. P.G. Coll, C. O'Sullivan and P.J. Browne, 'Lycanthropy Lives On', *British Journal of Psychiatry*, 1985, vol. 147, pp. 201–202.

70. *Independent*, 25 July 1987.

71. C.G. Jung, *Collected Works, Vol. 17*, London, Routledge and Kegan Paul, 1954.

72. Fahy *et al.* op. cit. 1988.

73. P.E. Keck, H.G. Pope, J.I. Hudson, S.L. McElroy and A.R. Kulick, 'Lycanthropy: Alive and Well in the Twentieth Century', *Psychological Medicine*, 1988, vol. 18, pp. 113–120.

74. See R. Littlewood, Letter, *British Journal of Psychiatry*, 1986, vol. 148, pp. 340–341.

75. See C. Wallis, 'Zombies – Do They Exist?', *Time*, 17 October 1983, p. 60.

76. See W. Davis, *The Serpent and the Rainbow*, London, Collins, 1986. It appears that ingestion of the puffer-fish (fugo/fuga pardalis), a favoured Japanese delicacy, can produce death if incorrectly prepared. The symptoms are said to be very similar to those demonstrated in cases of alleged Zombiism.

77. Notably his paper 'The Ethnobiology of the Haitian Zombi', *Journal of Ethnopharmacology*, 1983, vol. 9, pp. 85–104. Some of his neuro-pharmacological findings have been subjected to criticism by R. Wittes and his anthropological findings by E. Bourguignon, both in the *Journal of Transcultural Research*, 1985, vol. 22, pp. 191–194. (I am grateful to Dr K. de Pauw for bringing these papers to my attention.)

78. See Walker, op. cit. 1978, pp. 191–192.

79. See for example, S.M. Smith and J. Dimock, 'Necrophilia and Anti-Social Acts', in L.B. Schlesinger and E. Revitch (eds), *Sexual Dynamics of Anti-Social Behaviour*, Springfield, Illinois, Charles C. Thomas, 1983, Chapter 13.

80. Quoted in Favazza, op. cit. p. 7.

81. For a description of the Christie case see L. Kennedy, *Ten Rillington Place*, London, Gollancz, 1961, and, more briefly, Smith and Dimock, op. cit. 1983, p. 249.

82. Smith and Dimock, op. cit. 1983, pp. 248–249.

83. See B. Masters, *Killing for Company: The Case of Dennis Nilsen*, London, Jonathan Cape, 1985.

84. *Guardian*, 27 March 1985.

85. A.A. Bartholomew, K.L. Milte and F. Galbally, 'Homosexual Necrophilia', *Medicine, Science and the Law*, 1978, vol. 18, pp. 29–35.

86. N.P. Lancaster, 'Necrophilia, Murder and High Intelligence', *British Journal of Psychiatry*, 1978, vol. 132, pp. 605–608.

87. See postscript by Dr Anthony Storr at pp. 317–325.

88. Quoted in D.J. West, *Sexual Crimes and Confrontations: A Study of Victims and Offenders*, Aldershot, Gower, 1987, p. 179.

89. See, for example, R.M. Holmes and J. de Burger, *Serial Murder, Studies in Crime, Law and Justice, Volume 2*, London, Sage, 1988.

90. West, op. cit. 1987, p. 183.

91. M. Cox, 'Dynamic Psychotherapy with Sex Offenders', in I. Rosen (ed.), *Sexual Deviation* (2nd edn), Oxford, Oxford University Press, 1979, p. 310. See also A.H. Williams, 'The Psychology and Treatment of Sexual Murderers', in I. Rosen (ed.), *The Pathology and Treatment of Sexual Deviation*, London, Oxford University Press, 1964.

92. R.P. Brittain, 'The Sadistic Murderer', *Medicine, Science and the Law*, 1970, vol. 10, pp. 198–208.

93. Such planning was characteristic of the killings committed by David Berkowitz, the so-called 'Son of Sam' in the U.S.A. Over a period of about a year young women were shot dead; their boyfriends were also attacked and in some cases killed. There was no evidence of sexual molestation but an underlying sexual motive emerged. Berkowitz, at age 24, was, of course, younger than those depicted in Brittain's profile. But he did, however, show some of the ambivalent prudishness depicted in Brittain's account. He is said to have told a psychiatrist 'sex outside of marriage is a heinous sin'. He was also preoccupied by sexual phantasies, extremely shy with women and frightened that he might be impotent in sexual encounters with them. See West, op. cit. 1987, p. 185.

94. See Schlesinger and Revitch, op. cit. 1983, p. 214.

95. See H. Prins, *Dangerous Behaviour: The Law and Mental Disorder*, London, Tavistock, 1986, especially Chapters four and six.

96. See P.E. Igbinovia, 'Ritual Murders in Nigeria', *International Journal of Offender Therapy and Comparative Criminology*, 1988, vol. 32, pp. 37–43.

97. See in particular the very comprehensive treatment of this topic by Resnik in Schlesinger and Revitch, op. cit. 1983, Chapter 12.

98. Resnik, in Schlesinger and Revitch, op. cit. 1983, pp. 243–244.

99. B. Knight, 'Fatal Masochism – Accident or Suicide?', *Medicine, Science and the Law*, 1979, vol. 19, pp. 118–120.

100. S. Sivaloganathan, '*Curiosum Eroticum* – A Case of Fatal Electrocution During Auto-erotic Practice', *Medicine, Science and the Law*, 1981, vol. 21, pp. 47–50.

101. S. Sivaloganathan, *'Aqua-eroticum* – A Case of Auto-erotic Drowning', *Medicine, Science and the Law*, 1984, vol. 24, pp. 300–302.
102. N. Ikeda, A. Harada, K. Umetsu and T. Suzuki, 'A Case of Fatal Suffocation During an Unusual Auto-erotic Practice', *Medicine, Science and the Law*, 1988, vol. 28, pp. 131–134. For further illustration see cases described by S.M. Cordner in, 'An Unusual Case of Sudden Death Associated With Masturbation', *Medicine, Science and the Law*, 1983, vol. 23, pp. 54–56.

Chapter six

Concluding comments

'Here is my journey's end, here is my butt,
And very sea-mark of my utmost sail.'
(*Othello*, Act V, Scene ii)

The aim of this short book has been very modest. It has been to introduce readers to a range of somewhat idiosyncratically chosen unusual disorders of behaviour. One might well question what is to be gained from describing such behaviours and some may assert that a preoccupation with such rarities could be seen as morbid or prurient. There are cogent arguments against such assumptions. In the first place, the study of so-called extreme forms of behaviour can be useful in teaching us about the whole range of human conduct. In the second place, these behaviours have their counterparts in so-called 'normality'. For example, many of the disorders described in Chapter two seem to be but extensions of normal states seen in most people, a good illustration being that of jealousy. Even states of so-called 'possession' are not regarded as 'abnormal' in some cultures. Such a view reminds us of the importance of seeing some of the behaviours described in this book, most notably the so-called culture-bound syndromes, within a multi-disciplinary context.[1] As already suggested, this is becoming increasingly important in contemporary multi-cultural society. One of the most important lessons to be learned from some of the illustrations provided in this book is the influence of myth and legend in providing fertile ground for the manifestation of some kinds of highly unusual behaviour. This is perhaps best illustrated in the discussion of vampirism in Chapter five, and even the apparently grossly abnormal behaviour of the necrophile has to be seen within a historical and psychopathological context. For do we not expend a great deal of time and effort on beautifying the dead – and for a variety of reasons? I think we have a responsibility to search for meanings in behaviour, however unusual and unpalatable they may sometimes appear. I also think we can only do this if we pay careful attention to their complex origins. Some of my illustrations of some of these approaches, such as the attempts to explain vampirism through the discipline of forensic pathology, I hope will have demonstrated how useful such approaches can be. Finally, this book can be read in two ways. It can be seen as a useful introductory guide to certain unusual forms of behaviour and to this extent may be said to be self-contained. Those wishing to take each of the topics further will be greatly assisted by the wealth of detailed literature I have assembled in the 'Notes and references' at the end of each chapter, and in the section on 'Additional reading'. Such reading will provide material for a life-time's study of forms of behaviour that may not only 'beggar belief', but may uncomfortably raise the spectre of some of our innermost and barely recognised feelings and phantasies.

Note and reference

1. The need for such an approach has recently been argued very cogently by a distinguished professor of psychiatry, John Nemiah. In discussing psychiatric disorders he asserts that 'The basic unit of study for psychiatric investigation is the individual human being in interaction with the environment' (J.C. Nemiah, 'The Varieties of Human Experience', *British Journal of Psychiatry*, 1989, vol. 154, pp. 459–466).

Additional reading

Some of the works cited below are also referred to in the 'Notes and references' following each chapter, but they are included here because they contain material additional to the original reference.

Chapter one

M. Cox and A. Theilgaard, *Mutative Metaphors in Psychotherapy: The Aeolian Mode*, London, Tavistock, 1987. (Brings together clinical, literary and metaphorical material in a unique way).

A. Sims, *Symptoms in the Mind: An Introduction to Descriptive Psychopathology*, London, Baillière Tindall, 1988. (Especially Chapter 1.)

Chapter two

P. Bowden, 'De Clérambault Syndrome', in R. Bluglass and P. Bowden (eds), *Principles and Practice of Forensic Psychiatry*, London, Churchill Livingstone, 1990.

D. Enoch, 'Ganser Syndrome and Munchausen's Syndrome', in R. Bluglass and P. Bowden (eds), *Principles and Practice of Forensic Psychiatry*, London, Churchill Livingstone, 1990.

M.D. Enoch and W.H. Trethowan, *Uncommon Psychiatric Syndromes* (2nd edn), Bristol, Wright and Sons, 1979.

P. Mullen, 'Morbid Jealousy and the Delusion of Infidelity', in R. Bluglass and P. Bowden (eds), *Principles and Practice of Forensic Psychiatry*, London, Churchill Livingstone, 1990.

Chapter three

M. Martin, *Hostage to the Devil*, London, Bantam Books, 1977.

R. Parker, *The Occult: Deliverance from Evil*, Leicester, Inter-Varsity Press, 1989. (Especially Chapters 7–11.)

M.S. Peck, *People of the Lie: The Hope for Healing Human Evil*, London, Rider, 1988. (Chapter 5)

Chapter four

P. Bowden, 'Amok', in R. Bluglass and P. Bowden (eds), *Principles and Practice of Forensic Psychiatry*, London, Churchill Livingstone, 1990.

M. Lipsedge, 'Cultural Influences on Psychiatry', *Current Opinion in Psychiatry*, 1989, vol. 2, pp. 267–272.

R. Littlewood, 'From Categories to Contexts: a decade of the "new Cross-Cultural Psychiatry"', *British Journal of Psychiatry*, 1990, vol. 156, pp. 308–327.

R. Littlewood and M. Lipsedge, *Aliens and Alienists*, Harmondsworth, Penguin Books, 1982.

Chapter five

P. Barber, *Vampires, Burial and Death*, London, Yale University Press, 1988. (Especially Chapters 3, 11, 12 and 13.)

R. Bluglass, 'Bestiality', in R. Bluglass and P. Bowden (eds), *Principles and Practice of Forensic Psychiatry*, London, Churchill Livingstone, 1990.

C. Gosselin and G. Wilson, *Sexual Variations: Fetishism, Sado-masochism and Transvestism*, London, Faber and Faber, 1980.

S. Hucker, 'Sexual Asphyxia, Necrophilia and Other Unusual Philias', in R. Bluglass and P. Bowden (eds), *Principles and Practice of Forensic Psychiatry*, London, Churchill Livingstone, 1990.

L.B. Schlesinger and E. Revitch (eds), *Sexual Dynamics of Anti-social Behaviour*, Springfield, Illinois, Charles C. Thomas, 1983, Chapters 11–15.

M. Summers, *The Werewolf*, New York, University Books, 1966.

F. Wertham, *Dark Legend*, New York, Doubleday, 1950.

Index

maternal deprivation 78, 79, 87
Mawson, D. 20
Meadow, R. 21
media, influence of 43, 48, 76
Mellor, C.S. 61
Mellsopp, G. 20
memory disorders 15, 18, 84 *see
    also* amnesia
memory repression 18
mengamok 44
Menuck, M. 60
Merskey, H. 60
Mestrovic, S.G. 40
Milgrom, L. 96
Milte, K.L. 99
miryachit 57
Mitchill, S.L. 17, 22
Mongolia 57
Monkseaton killings 50–1
Morley, S.J. 62
Mullen, P.E. 20
multiple personality disorder 17–19,
    32
Munchausen's syndrome 12–14
Munro, A. 20
Munthe, Axel 19, 22
murder 75, 85–6, 87–90
Murphy, H.B.M. 60
mutilation 24, 77, 90
mysticism 30
myths and mythology 4, 65, 84, 90,
    101; and lycanthropy 80; and
    vampires and vampirism 68–72,
    73–4

Nandris, G. 98
Narayanan, H.S. 40
necrophagia 74, 76
necrophilia xi, 74, 76, 84–7, 101
necro-sadism 76
Nell, C.W.O. 62
Nemiah, J.C. 102
Neustatter, W.L. 64, 93
New Testament *see* Bible
Nicaragua 30
Nigeria 90
Nilsen, Dennis 86, 87, 89
North American Indians 30, 58

Nosferatu 78
nuns: possession by demons 28

O'Keefe, D.L. 39
O'Sullivan, C. 98
occult 25, 34, 75, 89
Ohnuki-Tierney, E. 40
Ojibwa Indians 58
Old Testament *see* Bible
olonism 57
oral sadism 78, 79
oral sex 77, 97n
Orda, R. 98
Osterreich, T.K. 39
Othello syndrome 9
'over-valued ideas' 8

pain, insensitivity to 34
Palmer, B. 41
Papua New Guinea 47, 68, 97n
paranoid disorders 8, 46, 78
pathological lying 12
Pattison, E.M. 40
Pelosi, A.J. 40
pengamok 44
penile retraction, fear of 52–6
Perry, M. 39
personality disorders 12, 15–19, 32,
    74, 75, 78, 79, 83, 86
pibloktoq (piblokto) 58
Pliny 85
poisons/poisoning 10, 83–4
Pope, H.G. 98
porphyria 73, 96n
Porter, R. 38
possession and possession states
    23–38, 46, 58, 80
Prince, M. 17, 22
Prins, H. 19, 22, 93, 96, 99
promiscuity 9, 53, 54, 55
pseudologia fantastica 12
pseudonite 44
psychic vampirism 71, 78
psychodynamics 18, 45, 46
psychological 'profiles' 87–8
psychose passionnelle 10
Pullinger, K. 96